# ACHIEVING WELLNESS THROUGH ARTHRITIS

How My Journey With Ankylosing Spondylitis
Can Offer a Path to Wellness

## Chris Pudlak

Foreword written by Dr. Kiran Manhas

Achieving Wellness Through Arthritis
Copyright © 2021 by Chris Pudlak

All rights reserved. No part of this publication may be reproduced, distributed, or transmitted in any form or by any means, including photocopying, recording, or other electronic or mechanical methods, without the prior written permission of the author, except in the case of brief quotations embodied in critical reviews and certain other non-commercial uses permitted by copyright law.

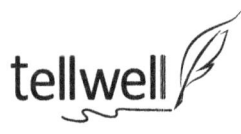

Tellwell Talent
www.tellwell.ca

ISBN
978-0-2288-4966-7 (Hardcover)
978-0-2288-4967-4 (Paperback)
978-0-2288-4965-0 (eBook)

How a journey with ankylosing
spondylitis can guide us to living well

Written by Chris Pudlak

"*One of the big bottlenecks in getting science translated into the real world is communicating to the public. There're many scientists that either avoid intentionally, or just don't want to bother with taking the time to learn how to communicate with the general public.*"

*Mark Mattson: Former Chief of the Laboratory of Neurosciences at the National Institute on Aging*

# CONTENTS

Dedication ..................................................................... xi
Foreword..................................................................... xiii
Preface ......................................................................... xv

**Chapter 1.  AS – A Summary................................................ 1**
A brief summary of AS: What is ankylosing spondylitis?........... 1
Comorbidities – complications of AS ....................................3
    Uveitis – eye inflammation ...............................................3
    Gastrointestinal Illness – inflammatory bowel disease..........4
    Plantar fasciitis and heel pain ...........................................5
    Synovitis (swelling/inflammation of the joint lining) ..........6
    Symptoms ......................................................................8
    Diverticulosis .................................................................8
Fatigue..............................................................................9
    Anemia........................................................................ 11
Expected medical treatments............................................. 14
    Antibiotics................................................................... 14
    Celecoxib .................................................................... 14
    Prednisone................................................................... 15
    Non-steroidal anti-inflammatory drugs (NSAIDs)
    and disease-modifying anti-rheumatic drugs (DMARDs) .. 15

**Chapter 2.  My Personal Experience With AS ..................... 16**
Cutting out naproxen.........................................................21
Cutting out sulfasalazine....................................................23
Personal symptoms that may have been
preliminary signs of AS .....................................................25
Tracking inflammation and blood markers ..........................28
    Enzymes in the blood....................................................28
    C-reactive protein.........................................................30

## Chapter 3. Medical Treatments ............................................. 32
TNFα suppression ................................................................. 33
COX-1/COX-2 suppression .................................................. 34
NSAIDs ................................................................................. 35
DMARDs .............................................................................. 37
Sulfasalazine ......................................................................... 37
Methotrexate ........................................................................ 39
Hydroxychloroquine ............................................................. 39
Biologics ............................................................................... 40
Steroids ................................................................................. 40
    Prednisone ....................................................................... 40
    Cortisone injections ........................................................ 42
Supplements ......................................................................... 43
Topical treatments ............................................................... 44
    Essential oils .................................................................... 44
    Diclofenac ....................................................................... 45
    Vagal nerve stimulation .................................................. 45
    Drug financial conflicts .................................................. 46

## Chapter 4. Causes ..................................................................... 48
Free radicals ......................................................................... 48
    Solutions to free radicals - antioxidants ........................ 50
    Preventive antioxidants - glutathione ............................ 50
    Isoflavones ....................................................................... 51
    Flavanols ......................................................................... 51
    Hydroxycinnamic acids .................................................. 51
    Scavenging antioxidants—vitamin C ............................ 52
    The final step in the strategy—fasting .......................... 53
Pro-Inflammatory Cytokines ............................................... 53
Epstein-Barr virus ................................................................ 55
Dietary starch and inflammation ........................................ 56
    Rapidly digested starch – simple starches and sugars ... 56
    Indigestible starches ....................................................... 57
    Resistant starch ............................................................... 57

Starch and Klebsiella ................................................................. 58
Is starch feeding a monster? ...................................................... 60
    Amylase supplementation ..................................................... 62
Inflammation, gut health perspective ......................................... 63
Digestive system health ............................................................. 64
Purging bacteria from the colon – an accidental
but telling experiment ............................................................... 65
Overeating ................................................................................ 67

## Chapter 5.   Klebsiella ....................................................... 71
Treatment by controlling Klebsiella ............................................ 71
Calculating starch ..................................................................... 72
Iodine testing your food for starch – Don't feed Klebsiella! ...... 72
Foods to avoid that feed Klebsiella ............................................ 75
Resistant starch in foods ............................................................ 76
Klebsiella bactericidals ............................................................... 84

## Chapter 6.   Fasting to Reduce Inflammation ................ 86
Cortisol ..................................................................................... 87
Ketone bodies ............................................................................ 87
Intermittent fasting: Incorporating fasting into your life .......... 89
Fasting for longer durations ...................................................... 92
    Feedback from my doctors ..................................................... 92
    Forty-hour fast ...................................................................... 93
    Extended fasts, three to seven days ........................................ 93
Body mass index ....................................................................... 95
Refeeding after fasting ............................................................... 98
    Best refeeding foods (organized by nutrient) ....................... 100
    Recommended meals for refeeding after a fast .................... 102
    Order to reintroduce foods .................................................. 102

## Chapter 7.   Anti-Inflammatory Foods and Diet ......... 105
Foods ...................................................................................... 106
    Nutrients – vegetables (all non-root veggies) ....................... 108

- Nutrients – animals ... 109
  - Fats ... 109
  - Protein ... 111
  - Carbohydrates (grains/nuts/seeds, other) ... 111
  - Carbohydrates (fruit) (generally all fruit are ok but in moderation due to sugar) ... 111
- Supplements ... 112
- Probiotics ... 114
- Foods in moderation ... 116
  - Vegetables ... 117
  - Oils ... 117
  - Proteins ... 118
  - Nuts, Grains, carbs ... 119
  - Fruit ... 121
  - Others ... 121
- Foods (and habits) to avoid: ... 122
  - Overeating ... 122
  - Inflammatory oils ... 123
  - Synthetics ... 124
  - Sugars ... 125
  - Foods that feed Klebsiella ... 126
- Nutritional labels ... 128
- Nutritional claims ... 131
  - Source of fibre ... 131
  - Low fat ... 131
  - Cholesterol-free ... 131
  - Sodium-free ... 131
  - Reduced in calories ... 132
  - Light ... 132
  - Polyunsaturated fats ... 132
  - Monounsaturated fats ... 133
- Polyunsaturated fats ... 133
  - Omega-3s ... 133
  - Omega-6s ... 134

Saturated fats ........................................................................ 138
Daily calories – food list ..................................................... 144

## Chapter 8. Diet ............................................................. 149
Protein restriction ................................................................ 152
Calorie restriction and total energy expenditure .................. 153
Specific carbohydrate diet, fermentation and FODMAP ....... 156
Gluten-free and lectin-free diet ............................................ 158
Low-starch diet ................................................................... 159
Ketogenic diet ..................................................................... 159
20:4 fasting, OMAD diet .................................................... 160
Alternate-day fasting ........................................................... 162

## Chapter 9. Mind and Muscle .................................... 164
Exercise ............................................................................... 164
    Swimming .................................................................... 166
    Rowing ......................................................................... 167
    Pilates ........................................................................... 167
    Stretching ..................................................................... 167
    Resistance exercises ..................................................... 168
    Cycling ......................................................................... 168
Mind and spirit ................................................................... 169
Circadian clock ................................................................... 172

## Chapter 10. General Management and Solutions ............ 176
What worked? What didn't?
(Assessment of treatment effectiveness) ................................ 176
    Clear positive benefits .................................................. 178
    Moderate positive benefits ........................................... 181
    Benefits Unknown/unclear ........................................... 183
    Clear negative effects ................................................... 185
Suspected cause of my AS .................................................... 188
Causes – root cause and corrective action ............................ 190
Health strategy .................................................................... 195

General diet strategy ........................................................ 195
Specific goals .................................................................. 195
Specific targets ............................................................... 196
Closing recommendations ............................................... 197

**Chapter 11. Recipes ................................................ 199**
Starch-free meal ideas ....................................................200
   Breakfast ...................................................................200
   Salads/snacks, lunches ...............................................207
   Mains ........................................................................ 218
   Desserts .....................................................................225
   Condiments ..............................................................233

Acknowledgements ........................................................ 245
Glossary of Abbreviations .............................................. 247
References ......................................................................249

# DEDICATION

This book is dedicated to my children. I hope this book will help them make good lifestyle choices. May this information on managing arthritis always be available to them in need, and may they never need it.

# FOREWORD

I have known Chris since 2016 when he was diagnosed with ankylosis spondylitis. As physicians, it is our role to support and educate our patients in understanding their diseases. In turn, each patient experience is unique and offers us an opportunity to learn from them. For Chris, receiving his diagnosis was life changing and initially overwhelming. But from the start, he was curious, questioning, observant and detailed in his journaling, which ultimately helped him to understand and accept what was happening to his body and provided a strong base to tell his story.

As an engineer, he brings a unique perspective on understanding his disease, often tackling it as an engineering problem, which no doubt reflects his desire to establish concrete solutions. However, it is important to keep in mind that direct links or connections between symptoms and causes can be very difficult to establish in medicine and are not often a linear relationship due to the complexity of a myriad factors in our body as a system. This book summarizes his reflections as he struggles to grasp what was going on to him, and should not replace medical advice and may not represent everyone's experience.

That being said, I believe that his story should be shared. I appreciate his efforts to touch on various solutions in the areas of diet, exercise and available medical treatments, all important aspects of managing any chronic health condition. A better understanding and awareness of rheumatic diseases, disease progression and treatment options is always beneficial and will help patients with their own understanding and involvement in decisions made with their medical team. In addition to the medical advice he received from his physicians, Chris also found the support and guidance from other patients invaluable to understanding and managing his disease. In fact, it was appreciation for this support which motivated him to write this book, hoping to share his story with as many patients as possible to help them in their own journeys.

If you are recently diagnosed with AS or another form of inflammatory arthritis, or have similar symptoms, I encourage you to read his story.

—Dr. Kiran Manhas

# PREFACE

## Why I wrote this book

In the summer of 2016, I was struck with a severe onset of a type of arthritis which was later diagnosed as ankylosing spondylitis (AS). At the onset and formal diagnosis of my AS, I needed two hands just to turn the key in my car ignition, I limped when I walked, was unable to sit for more than half-an-hour at a time, unable to ride my bike, unable to pick up my children and I couldn't sleep a full night without being woken up several times due to joint pain. I resorted to wrapping my wrists while I slept to keep them immobile; any motion would cause sharp pain and wake me up. I could only sleep on my back, with a pillow under my back and a pillow under my knees. Even the weight of the sheets on my toes caused enough pressure to make my feet get sore.

I decided to record my daily symptoms, medications taken, diet, changes in exercise and activity, my blood test results, and a pain rating on a scale of 10. It became so severe, so quickly, that from the onset of my condition, I logged my pain, medications, diet and habits in detail. This information gathering was initially for my own benefit; I hoped to better understand the condition and figure out what was causing it so I could be rid of it as quickly as possible, and at the time, had no idea my obsessive note taking would turn into a book.

It took me about a year and a half to claim a "recovery" from AS, to the point where I can thrive and live actively without medication. However, to this day I often feel the AS, not too deeply under the surface, and I still deal with daily pain, occasional flare-ups and persistent low-level back pain and stiffness. I had to make many lifestyle changes to keep the condition under control, and it's these changes that keep it under control. There is no known cure for AS, but it certainly can be managed to allow sufferers to live fully.

Through the actions I have outlined in this book, I have recovered all my past physical activities (cycling, swimming, playing with my kids, rowing, and even some light running). However, many setbacks and flare-ups have reminded me that I need to continue to practice what I preach to manage the condition daily and keep it under control. It has not gone away, merely subsided, but I can confidently say, managed. I have received various medications through the course of my treatment, and they helped with my recovery, but due to the long-term nature of the condition I was motivated to substitute medication with supplements, and eventually supplements with diet. Forty years of pills was just not an option for me and I was not going down that road if I could help it, especially considering that I was experiencing side effects after less than a year. Physiotherapy was also an important factor in recovery and led me to take up stretching and Pilates daily. Eventually this evolved to include a weight-lifting program that helped me build the muscle in my back and shoulders to better protect and support my joints. Maintaining good posture is also important when managing AS. Sitting on a Swiss ball and using a standing desk at work have been positive contributors to rebuilding strength in my back. In the long term, it will also prevent joints from fusing in awkward postures. Dieting also had a positive effect, by dropping inflammatory foods, stacking my diet with anti-inflammatory foods, and using fasting therapeutically to reduce inflammation. I eventually found research by Dr. Alan

Ebringer, investigating the possibility that *Klebsiella pneumoniae*, a bacterium in the gut, combined with a gene (HLA-B27, which I tested positive for and has a clear association with AS) is the trigger for the arthritic inflammation. Furthermore, the *Klebsiella* was fed by amylose starch. Once I cut this type of starch out of my diet, it also helped greatly and virtually eliminated all arthritic flare-ups, although a lower-level back pain was still persistent.

But why would I recommend this book to anyone? Of all the changes I made in my lifestyle, I can't count the number of times I told myself, These are changes I should be making anyway. Diet, exercise, patterns of eating, stress management, sleep habits were all things I should have been managing better before the onset of my AS. They are related to other diseases as well, including obesity, diabetes and cancer. This book is a summary of the information I collected and confirmed through experimentation with my own condition, to share my experiences to hopefully make it easier for others experiencing the same challenges.

## How to use this book

This book started as a guide for others suffering with ankylosing spondylitis, but it evolved into a path to wellness for friends and family that I hope to extend to more readers. The information in this book can be applied to other inflammatory autoimmune diseases, and even cancer, as my focus for management has heavily relied on diet and lifestyle changes that dealt with my AS on a fundamental level, addressing underlying root causes that can contribute to many illnesses. In the first chapter, I provide the reader with background information on the condition, and in chapter 2, my history with it, to provide a baseline comparison to the extent of their condition. I then discuss medical treatments in chapter 3, which is where I started with my own experience, before I understood other methods for controlling the condition and inflammation in general. Once I started to investigate the causes, discussed in chapter 4 and chapter 5, I was able to experiment and research and apply solutions involving fasting (chapter 6), diet (chapters 7 and 8) and stress management and exercise (chapter 9). With this information, I hope to provide enough information on treatment options to help the reader manage arthritis through natural means.

I also hope that the information in this book may be useful to practitioners involved in arthritis and other autoimmune diseases. While the information is based on my own experience, a sample size of one, it often corroborates existing theories or studies, providing my own experience as another data point to show that the management strategies in this book can be successfully applied to managing arthritis. I have maintained strict records of changes in diet, medication, and lifestyle to show their impact on my blood inflammation levels and pain levels using the Bath Ankylosing Spondylitis Disease Activity Index (BASDAI) to provide the most accurate correlations possible.

## A lack of information, misinformation

Most of the guides to managing arthritis that I have received through formal medical channels barely discuss many of the most effective management strategies I've implemented. In many cases, I feel that the emphasis was way off the mark, and there is a big opportunity here to help others educate themselves on strategies that are both effective and natural, with the lowest risk of side effects. This was my biggest motivator in writing this book. I had to discover so much by myself, through my own research, and through trial and error and enough determination to test another natural solution when the first nine had not worked, spending months or years in the process. Relying on medication was a path I chose to avoid as much as it was within my power, through a desire to be an active husband and father, and without having consequences of side effects from medication over the next (hopefully) 40 years of my life. This drive helped me double my efforts every time my pain got worse, and eventually come across effective solutions. This is what books are for. I have learned the hard way through experience, and now I hope to pass on the experience to others. However, I do not mean for this book to be a step-by-step instruction.

One thing I found is that there are many exercises, diets, foods, and eating patterns that are effective in reducing inflammation and ultimately managing arthritis. The most effective is the one you can do on a regular basis, with the methods that best suit your lifestyle, schedule, interests, and past times. One that you are willing and able to implement. I strongly advocate natural solutions, but I am not against prescription drugs either. They helped me recover to where I am today but resulted in several side effects that took over a year to recover from on their own. However, if you need medications to reduce joint swelling, avoid long-term joint damage, and get active again, so be it. But the sooner you can substitute these medications with natural solutions, the better it is for your long-term health.

How could I possibly know this information before I was diagnosed with AS? I wish I had been handed a book like this. And while most of the research I will reference existed before my personal case, I didn't have access to it, so I didn't know it was there. I didn't know how important it was to follow. Sometimes, unfortunately, we need a health crisis in our lives to act as a wake-up call to start living right. The great benefit for me now, is that it can help me keep AS at bay, and hopefully delay or prevent some of the common diseases of our time, such as obesity, diabetes, cancer or other autoimmune diseases. The benefit for me now, is that I can share this path with others.

## The engineering approach

I do not have a degree in medicine, I am not a doctor, and I am not a rheumatologist. I was not faintly aware of the study of rheumatology before the onset of my condition. What gives me the credibility to write about arthritis? Since June 2016 I have suffered from ankylosing spondylitis and recently realized I have suffered early symptoms since 1997. Therefore, I can provide a firsthand account of my personal experience. For over four years, I kept a daily log on my progress. By education, and by career, I am an engineer; my degree is in applied science. This experience has been an exemplary chance to apply the scientific studies I have researched. This is precisely what engineers do; we take valuable research conducted by scientists and apply scientific principles to solve real-world problems.

I have taken studies and some of my own hypotheses and tested them on myself, sometimes proving my guesses, and sometimes disproving them despite multiple efforts to make them work. In these cases, the results were the most valuable because they were repeatable with consistent results. They ruled out any personal bias because they went against my desired outcome (feeling better). For example, cashews were on the list of "special carbohydrate foods" that I hoped I would be able to eat (I must disclose a conflict of interest here, I just like eating cashews and I wanted them to be part of my diet), but repeated attempts to include them in my diet always contributed to flare-ups. I believe this to be caused by the resistant starch content, which fit the pattern of flare-ups I found in other foods. My sample size was always one (I was the only one involved in my own personal tests), but I always had published studies to go by that involved more statistically significant group sizes, either in vitro or in vivo (which also should be taken into consideration, because tests in a petri dish don't always work out the same as in the gut); sometimes I fit in the group that benefited from the study, sometimes not. Another example would be curcumin. While studies show benefit for some, I noticed none. This may be why medical practitioners are sometimes reluctant to talk about or recommend diet. Individuals can have an assortment of allergies or intolerance, and the same list of foods does not work for all people. Seeing a nutritionist for allergy testing can help narrow down the field, and in a way, this is what I did for myself. Therefore, elimination diets consistently prove to be an effective way to understanding your personal condition, because they identify problem foods for the individual. However, based on my personal results, and the repeating patterns I have read in case studies and various diets, there are lists of foods and lifestyle changes that will help most. Even a collection of case studies, or a review of published studies, can show trends and indicate foods that can be used to reduce inflammation and treat arthritis.

In fact, I would argue that I have a unique perspective on my approach to managing my own arthritis. Since I am not a doctor, or a nutritionist or a physiotherapist, I do not have the same preconceived notions on how disease should be managed. I started this adventure more naïve and unaware than the practitioners guiding me, but this also allowed me to be more open minded to alternative solutions.

How else does an engineer qualify to write about a medical topic? I cannot help but feel the approach to problem solving in engineering is fundamentally different than it is in the pharmaceutical industry. (I say the pharmaceutical industry, not the medical profession, to be fair. I have some excellent doctors that do so much more for me than push me into the next medication.) The pharmaceutical industry seems to push medications to relieve symptoms. The focus is always on symptoms and rarely the under lying root causes. In engineering, especially the field of quality engineering, we are trained to determine the root cause. When products fail, you ask why. You break apart your problem into manageable sized chunks. In the case of a problem, you determine the condition and action that caused the symptom, and then you ask again, why these came about. You dig and dig until you uncover the true root cause. Then you apply a corrective action, or a solution, to each cause that is within your power to change. This is what I did with my condition, in this book. And, as is typical in life, there is clearly more than one root cause contributing to the condition. As a result, I recommend taking a holistic approach to making these changes in your life and pursuing as many of these solutions as possible. This will attack your arthritis from every angle possible and hopefully put it into remission, as it has for me.

Another engineering type of strategy is the idea of sampling. In science, you would use the scientific method. Using a hypothesis based on a lot of good theory and brain work, a scientist would develop a study and test the hypothesis to see if it were true or not. In engineering, random sampling is common. I applied this strategy at many times, sampling and testing foods and exercises with no real hypothesis in mind. I experimented, observed, and waited for trends to appear. I then apply a hypothesis after the fact and test further to see if it holds true. This is a good, mutual strategy to be used with the more traditional scientific approach. It also frees my mind of bias when entering a problem; I am not testing a hypothesis to try and build a case that a certain drug or diet works.

Why else should you listen to my advice on managing arthritis? I disclose no conflict of interest; I have no drugs to sell, no benefit from the sale of certain foods, and no financial benefit from anything I promote in this book. Much of what I promote includes fasting, exercise and lifestyle changes which, if anything, save you money. The true purpose of my years of investigation has been to resolve my own arthritis symptoms, and now I would like to share as much as possible.

My daily work involves designing tools. But I always find that the contractors who use my tools daily are always the best resource for design; they consistently give me the feedback from the field to design better tools. I liken this process to my own experience with arthritis. I am in the role of the contractor, getting my hands dirty on a daily basis, testing the tool, using the tool, dealing with the shortcomings of the tool. I suffer through arthritis firsthand, daily. I wake up with the pain every morning, and diligently logged my missteps and progress. What helped, what hindered. This data, I hope, can be an effective way to improve the understanding of an arthritis like AS and its treatment, and can be used to pass these experiences to other patients of arthritis like me.

# CHAPTER 1

# AS – A SUMMARY

**A brief summary of AS: What is ankylosing spondylitis?**

Ankylosing spondylitis is a type of arthritis primarily affecting the spine and other major joints in the body. Inflammation occurs at the entheses, where the tendons or ligaments insert into the bone. This inflammation activates bone growth as the body tries to repair itself, and the new bone growth can create more inflammation in the tendon, causing a repeating cycle. If the inflammation is left untreated, the adjacent bones (primarily in the spine) can continue to grow and eventually fuse together, causing the spine to become rigid; this is also referred to as *bamboo spine*. Having a rigid spine leaves it susceptible to fracture, most often at the location of the new bone growth where it is the weakest. This can eventually lead to deformity, further inflammation, and further bone growth.

AS is considered an autoimmune disease, and a seronegative spondyloarthropathy, meaning the patient normally tests negative for the rheumatoid factor, distinguishing this type of arthritis from rheumatoid arthritis, and placing it in a group of spondyloarthropathies (SpA) including psoriatic arthritis and reactive arthritis.

With AS, something in the body has gone amiss, and components of the body's immune system start attacking the body's own cells. There are a few reasons this is believed to happen. HLA-B27, an antigen that is inherited, has been associated with AS since 1973. Therefore, this disease has a genetic component. It has also been recognized that there is an environmental component. As sufferers of this condition, this is where we need to place our focus, since our environment (the air we breathe, the water we drink and the food we eat) is within our control to change.

Current theory stands that this environmental component that contributes to the disease is a combination of diet, and exposure to bacteria in the colon called *Klebsiella pneumoniae*. My personal story corroborates this theory. I feel that these three conditions were present in my case at the onset of my symptoms, as I later tested positive for HLA-B27, had a highly inflammatory diet, and suffered from gastrointestinal illness, fever and flu-like symptoms, which is consistent with a *Klebsiella* infection, and I tested positive for other viruses that are associated with AS.

While HLA-B27 likely accounts for about 30% of the overall risk of developing AS, not all people with HLA-B27 will develop AS, and not all people with AS have the HLA-B27 gene. However, there is still a strong correlation between the disease and the gene. Scientists suspect that other genes can also contribute; this research is ongoing. At the time of the writing of this book, researchers have identified more than 60 genes that are associated with AS and related diseases. Among the newer key genes identified are ERAP 1, IL-12, IL-17, and IL-23. (José Francisco Zambrano-Zaragoza, Ankylosing Spondylitis: From Cells to Genes, 2013)

The environmental factor, such as a bacterial infection, was very clear in my case. While I had suffered from some lower-back pain and peripheral arthritis before I was diagnosed with AS, these problems were never severe or clearly associated with each other. But when I had a case of gastrointestinal illness, the onset of my AS was explosive, and required quick diagnosis and medication to get the condition under control. In retrospect, the low-level back pain and arthritis I had before my full-blown onset of AS was a sign of the underlying condition, and when the causative conditions all came together in the perfect storm, the disease reared its ugly head with full force. In the several years before the explosive onset of my AS, I did experience increasing back pain that also correlated to earlier incidences of gastrointestinal illness.

## Comorbidities – complications of AS

AS does not just affect the spine. Unfortunately, the inflammation occurring in the body can affect other areas as well. The pattern of joint involvement may be a distinguishing feature in AS, which is usually present in the lower back (sacroiliac joint or SI joint) and other major joints in the body. In my case, I suffered arthritis in the SI joint, with pain and stiffness extending through my entire back, my heels and toes, left knee, both wrists, and left index finger.

### Uveitis – eye inflammation

Uveitis is a form of eye inflammation that is commonly associated with AS. It can be sight-threatening by affecting the middle layer of the tissue in the eye wall (the uvea). Symptoms include redness, pain and blurred vision. Immunosuppressive therapies including biologics can be used to manage uveitis. Even though this is common (per the Spondylitis Association of America, as many as 50% of cases of SpA), I have so far not had any symptoms in my eyes.

## Gastrointestinal Illness – inflammatory bowel disease

Patients with SpA typically (per Spondylitis Association of America, again around 50% of cases) develop gastrointestinal (GI) symptoms after the appearance of joint symptoms. In my personal situation, GI symptoms came on immediately and sharply before the onset of arthritis symptoms, on several occasions. I had some history of GI symptoms before the onset of my AS, although most of the time I was able to chalk it up to bad dietary choices or too much drink. However, I would often suspiciously have diarrhea or even vomit when everyone else at the party was eating the same food with no issues.

Inflammatory bowl disease (IBD) itself is usually diagnosed on endoscopy; however, further tests can sometimes be needed if the inflammation is in the small bowel. Problems with the stomach may also be caused by non-steroidal anti-inflammatory drugs (NSAIDs), like naproxen, one of the very drugs used to treat AS. In my case, pantoprazole sodium was prescribed to decrease stomach acids.

In SpA, a relationship exists between gut and joint findings: chronic gastrointestinal lesions are associated with more advanced sacroiliitis, spondylitis, and peripheral arthritis. Remission of joint inflammation correlates with disappearance of gut inflammation and the persistence of joint inflammation is mostly associated with the persistence of gut inflammation. (Steven DiLauro, 2011) How true I found this in my own experience. Often, there was a clear relief in back pain immediately after the clearing of GI issues, and a gradual reduction in joint pain while a "normalization" of gut function was underway. AS shows many connections to our gut health, and this is the first of many AS-gut connections I will make in this book.

## Plantar fasciitis and heel pain

In my personal experience, heel pain has been a big part of my symptoms. Pain here is usually caused by some form of overuse. The other setting in which it is common is the seronegative forms of spondylarthritis, such as AS.

> "Treatment may be a problem, with pain persisting despite NSAIDS and proper insole padding. Treating this pain, including other localized intense inflammation such as dactylitis, is commonly treated with local cortisone injections."
>
> -Arthritis, Thompson, P.221-.

I seemed to experience the typical symptoms and treatments for my feet, receiving cortisone injections in my heels and in my second toe to reduce swelling due to dactylitis (sausage toe). The medication was effective in managing symptoms when they were severe, especially swelling, although pain remained after swelling subsided. After the medications, I was able to quiet these remaining flare-ups and pains, including those in the heel, through fasting, sufficient rest, and foot support and cushioning. Incorporating rest days into my schedule has been very beneficial, as I try to be active most days to manage my arthritis. I have had a history of heel pain and was diagnosed with flat feet early in life. I was always hard on my feet, engaging in running and cycling and kickboxing for a while, but old existing pains and injuries flared up significantly during my onset of AS. With inflammation markers running high in my body, it seemed to ignite these old problems as well. It took a good six weeks off my bike to resolve the remaining pains, and since then I have been able to return to activity in moderation. Pains have crept back, but sufficient rest days after activity have helped keep pain and swelling at bay.

## Synovitis (swelling/inflammation of the joint lining)

One area of peripheral arthritis that developed during the onset of my AS was inflammation in the form of swelling, redness, warmth, pain, and stiffness in the ball of my right foot. I had a hammer toe develop, eventually on both feet, and it was one of the last areas to clear up with lasting deformity. It was difficult to manage because the recommendations for plantar fasciitis typically require rest, but I felt better with movement to address the arthritis. In fact, when I started taking a break from cycling and giving it a rest, icing it felt worse at times. I even received a cortisone injection in this location, which alleviated much of the swelling, but did not clear up the pain, as I probably still had tissue injury that I kept injuring in my daily cycling routine. I suspected this was both the AS, and the foot swelling as a symptom of an overuse injury, overlapping each other. I decided I would need to treat the foot swelling first, and gave myself prolonged rest. After about three weeks, swelling and inflammation was reduced, although throughout the three weeks the arthritis-type pain remained. By the end of the three weeks, the joint felt the same as my other arthritis-affected joints, showing the most pain and stiffness in the morning, and easing with activity. With the injury healed, I was able to ease back into my cycling routine and get the regular activity I needed to manage the arthritis.

Methods I used to address the plantar fasciitis and synovitis in the toe:

Rest and ice: Staying off the foot and applying ice packs help reduce the swelling and pain. I iced typically for 20 minutes at a time, twice a day.

Taping/splinting: I developed hammer toe in the second left toe, and taping the toe down actually provided a lot of benefit. It seemed to pull the toe down and flat into its normal position and alleviated the pressure on the inflamed joint behind the second toe (metatarsophalangeal joint). Research also shows that in severe synovitis, it can prevent drifting of the toe out of its normal position.

Stretching: With the cycling, I would commonly have tight calf muscles, which also seemed to affect other tendons in the foot such as the Achilles tendon and the plantar fascia. Daily stretching helped all these areas, including the toe.

Supportive shoes: I changed my shoes both in the house and at work. At home, in the past, I would always walk barefoot or in socks, but I decided to get a soft and flexible, flat pair of runners dedicated for use around the house, like slippers but with better support. These helped immensely in giving the joint the protection it needed to heal. At work, I sadly put away my favourite pointed-toe, heeled dress shoes (a style that I loved to wear but most definitely contributed to foot problems), and got myself a comfortable pair of office shoes, with a flat profile (no heel) and a large toe box, to give my toes room to rest in their natural positions.

Arch supports: I used these initially but transitioned away from them, because they tended to raise my heel, which I felt was part of the problem. Having had foot problems for over 20 years, I also tried custom orthotics that did not raise the heel, which were beneficial, but I feel like without the right shoe, they don't address the true problems (insufficient cushioning, insufficient toe space and width, and a heel that is too high). Combined with shoes that don't provide enough space, even custom orthotics can cause the additional problem of too much compression against the arch, which can cause numbness, and tendon rubbing, and prevent the arch from building its own supportive strength. I later went back to using a padded insert when I started running to add more impact protection.

Metatarsal pads: These distribute the weight away from the metatarsal joint. I had some moderate success with this, but it seemed to work best as a temporary solution to allow me to keep walking when swelling was at its worst. Once swelling and pain was manageable, I discontinued the use of pads and relied on correct shoes, resting to allow it to heal, and stretching and exercises to allow the foot to recover and strengthen.

## *Symptoms*

The symptoms that allowed me to identify this type of inflammation as synovitis included:

- Pain, particularly on the ball of the foot. It can feel like there is a rock under the ball of my foot, which can make it very difficult to walk. I would often limp or walk with my toe pointed inward, so my weight was on the outside of the arch and away from the swollen second toe.
- Swelling and pain, including the base of the toe.
- Pain when walking barefoot.

## *Diverticulosis*

This is a condition where pockets form in the intestinal wall, and the biggest risk with this is that food can become stuck in these pockets and cause an inflammatory condition called diverticulitis. This is not a feature of AS, but it raised a red flag when discussing AS with my mom. She told me that she has diverticulosis. Seeing as how ankylosing spondylitis already shows a link to intestinal health and diet, I suspected this may also be a contributor. My mother had a colonoscopy performed, so she was sure of her condition. I have had no such diagnosis, and this is not typically part of arthritis, but I couldn't help but think about the sensitivity of my gut and if this was a compounding factor. If you have gut problems, it may be worth investigating in your case.

## Fatigue

It is well known that ankylosing spondylitis can cause fatigue. The fatigue is generally understood to be caused by the inflammation occurring in the body. This seems to align with my own experience, as I had the most amount of fatigue when my C-reactive protein (CRP) readings were the highest, and when I was feeling the most joint pain. At the height of my symptoms, I just needed extra time to rest. A nap during the day, when I had the time, was a big help. However, too much rest, especially a deep sleep with absence of movement, would cause my back to stiffen up and make matters worse when I awoke. It was difficult to sleep for a normal duration because I would stiffen up so much. As my inflammation markers gradually came down, my fatigue also came down. Over the course of my condition, I found there were other causes that I could manage that would help reduce fatigue. They fell into a few categories: reducing medication, bad dietary practices, mistakes when adjusting to a healthier diet, and fasting.

I was trying very hard to reduce my dependence on medication, and while this was a good thing, I noticed a clear correlation to fatigue while weaning off various medications. Weaning off a very high dose of prednisone resulted in fatigue. Weaning off prednisone when phasing in sulfasalazine was typically associated with more severe pain and fatigue. Weaning off naproxen was also associated with an increase in pain and fatigue.

Bad dietary practices, including high glycemic index (GI) foods, also contributed to fatigue. Breaking my diet with a cinnamon roll or other high-GI food, overeating, eating a large meal, and having insufficient water intake would all result in fatigue.

Making mistakes while I was adjusting to a healthier diet caused fatigue. Moving to a keto diet led to insufficient calorie intake. For a while, I dropped 15 to 20 lbs in weight while I was adjusting to new eating patterns. Increasing the fat in my diet to obtain sufficient calories helped, and I felt better once I was at a stable weight. I was used to getting my calories from bread, pasta, and cereals, and for a while I did not know what to eat. I tried cutting out my daily coffee, just to see if I still had the will power to do so! Thankfully, I have never seen any negative correlations with consuming coffee, so I have kept it in my diet. I have experienced fatigue after transitioning back to a keto diet and I presume this is the body's response after consuming easy to use sugar stores and transitioning back to ketosis.

As I incorporated fasting into my routine, I also found it could cause fatigue. Extended fasting and transitioning to longer intermittent fasting (IF) seemed to cause fatigue, mostly related to insufficient water intake. Once I got used to IF, it became my preferred eating routine and did not cause me fatigue; even a 22-hour daily fast caused me no fatigue. My first three-day fast caused a notable "keto flu" during a trip back from Illinois. However, subsequent fasts did not cause the same fatigue, as my body got used to them. Another source of fasting-related fatigue was remaining inactive during the fast. I can always successfully break the fatigue by pushing myself to get active. So much of the fatigue from fasting is psychological. I can be in a really low-energy state, feeling like I have a slow metabolism and having cold hands when I'm working at my desk, but once I get on my bike and get moving, energy returns full strength.

In general, large meals, high-GI meals, transitioning off medication, and transitioning on to a keto diet all contributed to fatigue. One of the known side effects of ketosis is adrenal fatigue, and this generally happens when the body is transitioning from burning glucose to producing ketone bodies and burning fat. That initial drop in blood sugar, before the body can adjust, is the source of the fatigue. Once on a stable ketogenic diet, swings in blood sugar are reduced and so is fatigue. I liken this to cutting coffee. Weaning the body off caffeine can cause fatigue and headaches, but once the body adjusts, you have fewer highs and lows in energy.

I most often felt fatigued after a big meal, especially of foods with a high glycemic load. How did I solve this? Sticking to a moderately sized meal with lower glycemic load foods seemed to do the trick. Fatigue came way down. When transitioning to a keto diet, I found taking a tablespoon of medium-chain triglyceride (MCT) oil at wakeup (or even omega-3 supplement capsules), seemed to help a lot with my morning bike ride to work. But after a while, even this was not needed.

## Anemia

Anemia can be a characteristic finding of a chronic inflammatory disease such as AS. Anemia, in the case of AS, is usually normocytic (normal-sized hemoglobin) as the body cannot make blood as well in the setting of chronic inflammation. A microcytic anemia (small blood counts) can be seen in iron deficiency states, which can happen with chronic blood loss from inflammatory bowel disease, decreased iron absorption or poor dietary intake.

My blood results showed that I was anemic. Anemia can also cause fatigue. I was prescribed iron supplements to bring my iron levels up to normal levels; however, I was eventually able to improve my diet and phase out the iron supplements by getting enough iron in my food. On one side, I worked to increase the intake of iron-rich foods (such as liver, eggs, spinach, artichokes, lean meats, and seafood) and foods rich in cofactors (such as vitamin B6, folic acid, vitamin B12, and vitamin C) to maintain normal hemoglobin levels. I kept it in mind to select anti-inflammatory foods wherever possible, and to avoid starchy foods that could cause flare-ups:

- Foods high in iron include liver, clams, spinach, broccoli, nuts (in moderation, be aware of omega-6 levels) and seeds. Beans are also high in iron, but I do not recommend them due to starch content that may cause a flare in AS.
- Foods high in B12 include fish, especially oysters, sardines, organ meats, beef, clams, and nutritional yeast.
- Foods high in B6 include fish and vegetables in general.
- Foods high in folic acid, which aids in iron absorption, include broccoli, Brussels sprouts, liver, and spinach.
- Foods high in vitamin C, which aids iron absorption, including vegetables like bell peppers.

The other strategy to improve iron levels is to avoid foods that prevent iron absorption, such as food with tannins, like black tea, green tea, rooibos tea, coffee, grapes, wine, sorghum, and corn (which should be avoided for the starch anyway). Cut coffee? This is something I just could not do. Fortunately, you do not have to avoid these foods completely; you just need to avoid combining them with a meal containing iron, because when combined, tannins can interfere with iron absorption. The other ingredient to avoid is calcium, which can also interfere with iron absorption in a similar fashion. Do not remove calcium from your diet; just remember to consume it at separate times from iron.

As an engineer, antioxidants make me think of oxidation, and oxidation reminds me of rust on steel, and steel is mostly made up of iron. I could not help but wonder, does anemia, or the iron stores in the body in general, influence oxidative stress in the body? It turns out it does. One study treated patients with iron deficiency anemia by using six weeks of iron supplementation. It showed a significant decrease of oxidative stress in the body. (Kurtoglu E1, 2003) Again, we are seeing the relationship between comorbidities that exist with AS, but also that influence AS, which reinforces the need to take a holistic approach to identifying and addressing the causes.

If you have anemia like I did, get your iron stores up, get more energy for exercise and activity, and reduce the oxidative stress occurring in your body through iron to work together with other antioxidants in your diet. The reduced oxidative stress reduces inflammation and reduces AS symptoms to give you more freedom to move and strengthen your body. Moving around, stretching, building muscle to protect and support the joints, and performing resistance training to increase cellular AMPK levels to reduce chronic inflammation all help to reduce AS symptoms and produce a positive feedback loop. This is a synergistic approach that will help you tackle AS from multiple angles and increase your chances at recovery.

It also should be noted that a small protein called TNFα plays a major role in anemia. It inhibits iron release from the reticuloendothelial system (the body system that removes dead or abnormal materials from the body). The same high levels of TNFα that contribute to AS can also contribute to anemia. A study on the effects of anti-TNFα therapy showed an improvement in hemoglobin levels (Ki-Jo KIM, 2012), so it could be presumed that foods that reduce TNFα levels can also help anemia in AS patients.

## Expected medical treatments

There are several medications that are commonly used to manage AS. The front line drugs being NSAIDs (Non-steroidal Anti-inflammatory Drugs), steroids such as prednisone or local cortisone injections, and DMARDs (disease-modifying anti-rheumatic drugs). The strategy behind these drugs is usually to reduce inflammation, inhibit the COX-2 enzyme, or inhibit TNFα proteins. However, this is not the only part of the immune system that is involved and targeted in AS. Biologics, DMARDs made from genetically engineered proteins, target other parts of the immune system such as interleukins IL-17 in the body (a pro-inflammatory cytokine). Later in this book you will see that many foods or lifestyle changes use the same strategy to reduce inflammation, but typically to a lesser effect. In my case, I was prescribed antibiotics, celecoxib, prednisone, naproxen, cortisone injections (to treat dactylitis), sulfasalazine and methotrexate.

### Antibiotics

I had antibiotics prescribed to me during the onset of my symptoms. My GP had suspected septic arthritis or some other infection as the cause of my pain. Right around this time, I tested positive for the Epstein-Barr virus. Antibiotics are usually not part of the traditional management of AS.

### Celecoxib

This was one of the first medications I received during the initial onset of my AS. I felt no benefit at that stage, but perhaps the condition was too strong for the medication because soon after, I was being prescribed increasingly large doses of prednisone, a potent steroidal drug.

*Prednisone*

Prednisone is a powerful, steroidal, anti-inflammatory drug. When it was prescribed in my case, it was highly effective in countering severe inflammation. However, the side effects were also significant, and discontinuing the drug could not be done immediately; I needed to be weaned off the medication over a period of about four weeks.

*Non-steroidal anti-inflammatory drugs (NSAIDs) and disease-modifying anti-rheumatic drugs (DMARDs)*

Naproxen is a common NSAID prescribed for arthritis. Often, proton pump inhibitors (PMIs) are prescribed with them to reduce stomach acid levels and reduce risk of side effects such as stomach ulcers. Common DMARDs include sulfasalazine, methotrexate, infliximab and adalimumab. The DMARDs antagonize TNFα proteins, which results in a dampening of the body's natural inflammatory response. Through researching diet, I've learned that many foods provide anti-inflammatory benefit through the same or similar pathways, targeting TNFα, inhibiting COX-1/COX-2, or suppressing the HLA-B27 gene or other proteins involved in inflammation, just like the medications. This similarity between medication and food motivated me to start working toward a transition—from treatment from medication to supplements, and from supplements to diet—to control my condition.

# CHAPTER 2

# MY PERSONAL EXPERIENCE WITH AS

My younger years were typical. High school, track and field, a university career filled with sometimes too much partying, sometimes too much work, but eventually managing to find a balance. When I was in university, between kickboxing and running, I had managed to develop Achilles tendonitis. I was always active, mostly with running and cycling. When I moved to British Columbia with my wife, I added a few activities to my list including hiking and snowboarding. Once we started having kids, of course life changed and became much busier. I managed to keep up the biking by biking to work on a regular basis. This was the best way for me to fit it in to a busy schedule. I still liked to run and would do trail running and the occasional 10k race. I enjoyed the running, but occasionally, I managed to give myself a slow-healing injury, usually in the ankle or heel area. I had a history of it.

For me, AS started quite suddenly. It was the summer of 2016; I was 36 years old. I was returning from a trip from Europe. My wife and three kids were travelling together, but I had been unsure of obligations with work, and by the time I was able to book my flight, there were no more seats available on my family's flight, so I was travelling back to Canada on my own. Maybe that was a good thing. They had a good flight back; mine was one of the worst I have ever experienced. I had to make several connections through the United States. My initial flight was delayed, so I missed my connection. I was rebooked on a flight from Dallas to Vancouver, departing at 9:00 p.m. local time. The plane was late arriving in Dallas, and when it did, it was announced that the crew had logged too many flight hours in the day and the next flight had to be cancelled until 6:00 a.m. the next day. Since it was already 11:30 p.m., all passengers had to sleep on cots at the gate. I already was not feeling well, and I had a horrible sleep. I had back pain and stomach cramps that night. I slept on the floor for about an hour until they brought us cots. When I arrived in Vancouver in the morning, I took a cab straight to work. I did not want to fall behind on another day of work. A second wind carried me through the day, but then everything took a turn for the worse.

High fever, diarrhea, and increased back pain continued over the next five days. And then, what I suspected to be gout flared up in my right big toe. I went to the closest clinic that was open over the weekend, and they also suspected gout. The next day, I was able to meet with my family doctor, and by then my back pain had increased, and my left knee was flaring up. My family doctor didn't think it looked like gout at this point, but she scheduled me for a blood test for gout and septic arthritis. Over the next couple days, the pain increased, and severe wrist pain was added to the list. I was prescribed celecoxib and cyclobenzaprine. From 15 days from onset, the pain had become so severe that it kept me up at night. I began seeing a physiotherapist and was prescribed 25 mg of prednisone, a corticosteroid, along with an antibiotic. The prednisone gave me the first bit of relief, but it was short-lived. A call from my doctor indicated that my CRP was 28.8 mg/L, my RH factor was negative, and I had sclerosis in the sacroiliac joint. My fever, chills and weakness continued, and I felt like I must have some type of infection. My next CRP reading, about 10 days later, was 42.5 mg/L, approximately double the previous reading.

I was prescribed an increase in prednisone from 25 mg to 50 mg a day. Again, it gave me some immediate relief. I was even able to take my kids to the airshow the next day, and I did some light but urgently needed renovation work around the house. Again, the relief was short-lived.

My next barrage of blood test results showed I was Hepatitis A or B negative, negative for Lyme disease, but I tested positive for the Epstein-Barr virus, which causes mononucleosis, but it was difficult to tell how long ago this infection had occurred. I couldn't handle the prednisone dosage for more than five days. Unfortunately, pain was increasing again, and I started noticing some moderate and frequent heart palpitations. I spoke with my doctor and went back to the 25 mg dosage. At this point, I was near my worst. My wrists were so sensitive, I could barely turn the key in the ignition of my car. Sitting in the car, and at work, was excruciating, but the worst of it was at night. I was sleeping with a pillow under my back, one under my knees, and my wrists wrapped in tensor bandages because any movement would result in sharp pain. I could forget about getting rest to help with recovery.

Chills, nausea, and mild fever continued, and I finally decided I had to do whatever else was in my power to help my condition. I decided to cut out processed foods and foods with added sugars, and I thought to try curcumin (an active ingredient in turmeric) because I heard it could help with inflammation. Now almost six weeks into my illness, I had my first appointment with a rheumatologist. She confirmed my condition was a type of spondylarthritis, most likely AS or reactive arthritis. She instructed me to start sulfasalazine and said that I should see results in one to three months. I was also to wean off the prednisone over a period of four weeks. I was happy about that; I didn't think my heart could take much more of it. On top of it all, I could take 1,000–1,500 mg of ibuprofen per day (I was already taking about half that daily). As I reduced the prednisone dosage, things got a little worse before they got better, but my joints, fever, nausea, and diarrhea gradually did get better over the next three months. Between the physiotherapy, sulfasalazine, diet changes, naproxen, and the prednisone I was still taking in reduced amounts, something (or everything) was slowly helping. Joint pain moved around between my toes, heels, balls of my feet, left knee, lower back, and wrists.

And on top of the pain was the fatigue. A blood test was now showing that I was anemic, so I was prescribed 300 mg of ferrous gluconate per day. The good news was that my CRP was back down to 23.4 mg/L; still very high, but at least trending downward. I had phased off the prednisone, now two-and-a-half months into my illness.

I was making very slow but gradual progress. Day-to-day, I didn't notice any change, but over the weeks, by logging my progress, I noticed an improvement. However, I soon ran into another problem with my foot. I stubbed my foot climbing the stairs one afternoon. Since my left-hand toe was stiff from the arthritis, it took the brunt of the impact. It immediately turned black and blue, and swelled up like a sausage. I'd stubbed toes before, but this time it was a severe, over-reactive inflammatory response from the injury. I was still suffering enough at night for my knee or back to wake me up and the pain was intolerable without a pillow holding them both in a neutral position. However, I was eager to get active again, and ready to try cycling and swimming. Cycling was hard. Every little bump was horribly jarring on my wrists. A 15-minute session of swimming was much easier on the joints, but I went back to feeling sore and tight soon after. I tried to keep it up without overdoing it, as I was told that activity is good for AS. Cortisone shots at this point were a big benefit, starting with four shots in my toes. The next day my left foot was feeling better, and I had a good gradual improvement over the next week. I tried swimming and biking again, but biking was very tough on the knee.

I was now three-and-a-half months into my illness and starting to see good weekly improvements. I couldn't do a full squat, but range of motion in my knee was improving. I made three gentle bike rides in a week. I had occasional worsening of symptoms, but overall, the gradual trend was improvement. Five months from onset, my CRP was 12.4 mg/L, but my rheumatologist still recommended going from four tablets of sulfasalazine per day to six, and provided naproxen in place of ibuprofen, with pantoprazole sodium to protect my stomach from damage. I was keeping up the biking three to four times per week. I was still having some occasional heart palpitations and was worried this was somehow related to the naproxen. For the first time, I felt ready to reduce my naproxen dosage from four to two tablets per day. I held out for six days before an increase in pain convinced me to return to four tablets of naproxen per day. I gave myself another month before I tried again. I was up to biking five or six days per week, and my hands were strong enough to do a few chin-ups at a time. I also doubled down on my efforts to cut out processed (packaged) foods and foods with any added sugar. This time I was able to hold the reduced dosage of naproxen for about 15 days before I had to go back to the higher dosage. Again, I gave it another month, now seven-and-a-half months from onset. My CRP was down to 5.6 mg/L, and my rheumatologist provided me with cortisone shots in my left index finger.

Now 11 months since onset, most of the pain was in my feet, with some in my back and knee. I was gradually extending my rides to 30 km per day and five days per week. And then I hit a big milestone; I was able to bend my toes! I didn't have full range of motion yet, but the joint was popping occasionally, and I had most range of motion back, similar to the progress I experienced with my knee. After 11 months of limited mobility, this felt great. I felt ready to try to reduce my naproxen again. By this time, I was implementing intermittent fasting and calorie restriction: no sugar, limited carbs, no alcohol (which I had avoided since the onset of my condition), lots of fish, mussels, vegetables, chia, and green tea. A few days later, I tried my first day without any naproxen at all. I couldn't make it more than two days, but I felt the intermittent fasting was helping and I was encouraged to keep trying. My newest blood test helped with my motivation; my CRP was down to 0.9 mg/L! I doubled down on my efforts and believed my diet and activity efforts were helping. In a couple more weeks, I added omega-3 capsules to my diet and tried reducing my naproxen to one tablet per day. Now a full year after onset, I was trying to replace my naproxen as much as possible with omega-3s, intermittent fasting, a low-carb diet, exercise, and physiotherapy. This whole time, I was still taking six tablets of sulfasalazine per day. On the rare occasion, I could go a few days without naproxen, but I always had to go back to taking it for a short stretch to manage some occasional flare-ups.

## Cutting out naproxen

My effort to cut out naproxen ended up being very telling. For the first time, I started to notice an association between certain foods, activities, and pain flare-ups. My rheumatologist's strategy was to wean me off prednisone to clearly see how the disease was progressing and if I would respond to sulfasalazine (aside from the fact that prednisone has clear risks for long-term usage). Similarly, I felt like the naproxen covered up what was really going on with my diet, and that I needed to deal with some pain and flare-ups to understand how to improve my lifestyle. Fatigue was also apparent the more I cut naproxen, and I started to feel how overeating, or eating certain foods, was affecting my energy levels. Fatigue can be a sign of inflammation in the body; however, I believe this was, at least in part, caused by dietary changes (fatigue seemed to start when I significantly cut carb consumption, but resolved when I made an increase in dietary fat and balanced protein appropriately).

I researched diets, and gradually transitioned between a few of them. My low-carb and intermittent fasting (IF) strategy was initially focused on trying to achieve ketosis to help my natural cortisone levels. Once I learned about *Klebsiella* bacteria as a possible cause of AS, I increased my efforts to reduce carbs. I felt like this helped reduce pain, and I was able to discontinue naproxen entirely. However, it didn't help with fatigue. I lost 20 lbs and felt like I finally cut out 90% of my arthritis pain—this time without naproxen—but my energy levels were suffering. Plus, I really missed pizza, pasta, and cereal, which had always been the staples of my diet. Cooking became a new passion. In my research on *Klebsiella*, I learned a lot about starch, and how starch feeds these bad bacteria in the gut. There are also numerous studies that suspect biomimicry as the mechanism for *Klebsiella* to cause AS through the HLA-B27 antigen.

At this point, I learned of the Specific Carbohydrate Diet (SCD), first developed by Dr. Sidney Hass in the 1920's. This is when I realized that simple sugars like fructose and glucose are easily digestible carbs (monosaccharides) and it's the complex carbs that I really need to avoid. I was ready to start reintroducing foods to test my reaction to them, and many of these worked out fine, including most fruits like apples, or even raisins, which I initially feared would cause a problem due to their sugar content. Cashews were on the safe list in the SCD, and I like cashews, so despite them being relatively high in inflammatory omega-6, I repeatedly tried to reintroduce them into my diet. Unfortunately, they always caused a flare-up reaction. I finally came to understand this might be due to the resistant starch content, so I tested this idea. I started eating some carbs like naan bread (a traditional Indian flat bread) that I knew was low in resistant starch. It caused no flare-up, while otherwise healthy foods like cashews, caused a reaction. I felt like I had found the last piece of the puzzle.

Over the next several weeks, I tested and reintroduced foods with varying levels of success. Some had no effect, some had a very clear negative effect, but it was still difficult to determine the exact ingredient or method of preparation that caused the flare-up, especially when restaurant food was involved. This was especially true 15 months after onset, in October, when I had to travel for work for a week. I still prepared my own meals when possible, but restaurant meals with my co-workers most often caused flare-ups. When I was eating well, I could even tolerate a nine-hour day of driving; that amount of sitting would have been impossible a year before. But the mornings after a dinner at a restaurant, with foods not on my safe list, my back would flare up and it would take me an extra half hour in the morning to get loosened up and out of my hotel room. I managed to stay off the naproxen. The most effective method for bringing the flare-up under control was diet and activity.

Interestingly, during my week-long work trip, I found symptoms flared up considerably after experimenting with some restaurant foods that I hoped were sufficiently low enough in resistant starch. Once I began to return to my regular diet, I found some moderate reduction in my back flare-up, but the most noticeable difference was after I reintroduced a probiotic (kefir water, kefir and kombucha) after not having any probiotic food for the entire trip. Over the next few days back on my usual diet and exercise, my back and feet joint pain disappeared again.

## Cutting out sulfasalazine

One year and three months after the onset of my symptoms, I finally decided to try to cut out sulfasalazine. My rheumatologist recommended I take it for another two months, but I was concerned with some neck gland swelling that may have been a side effect of the medication. I felt I was ready, so with her approval

I cut it out. Initially, it had no effect. But after one month, I felt increasingly sensitive to eating the wrong foods that could result in flare-ups. Looking back at my log, I notice I was able to avoid arthritis pain flare-ups only when I was extra strict with my diet and careful to avoid starch. I feel the sulfasalazine helped, as it was more of a struggle to avoid flare-ups without it, but this was a challenge I chose to take so I could avoid taking the medication. I was preparing myself for the long haul, and I decided I didn't want to depend on medication for the next 40 years of my life if I could help it. In this process, I was careful to manage my pain based on what I could handle but avoid swelling because that was when joint damage would occur.

When I was cutting out naproxen, it had still acted as my fall back when flare-ups occurred or pain increased. I would try cutting naproxen out, hold out for a while on a new diet plan, but the pain would increase, and I would have to take some naproxen for one to four weeks to calm down my arthritis and give myself a chance to double my efforts on diet and try cutting naproxen again. Once I cut out sulfasalazine, fasting became my fall back technique for getting symptoms in check. Now, when my diet has gone awry, or even if I'm sore from biking and the arthritis is flaring up, I will fast—usually 36 hours does the trick—and it clears up everything quite nicely and it gives me a chance to get back into a clean diet. On top of that, I use 18- or 21-hour daily fasting as a daily maintenance tool and the occasional, three- to four-day fast when I feel a need for a deeper reset. I let my body tell me how long to go; usually a longer fast will feel therapeutic, not like a struggle, as if that's what my body needs. Fasting continues to be my strongest medicine and helps clear things up while I'm using tools like diet, exercise and stretching.

That gland pain in my neck that I noticed when I first started cutting out sulfasalazine never completely went away. It eased off for a while, but it transformed into a neck stiffness and soreness that seemed to become part of the arthritis associated with my back and the temporomandibular joint (TMJ) disorder in my jaw. While the remaining peripheral arthritis—mainly in my feet—dwindled away, the arthritis in my back, neck, and chest persisted and at times, worsened. With activity, stretching, and diet, I was able to keep it manageable, usually no more than a nuisance. A lot of physical activity (while being careful to avoid impact injury or overuse injury) was beneficial. A sore neck was helped by push-ups, shoulder exercises and weights. Daily stretching and Pilates helped my entire back. Light and careful eating was always beneficial. At one point I was feeling good enough to risk some starch and tried introducing red kidney beans, only to have a mild but very noticeable, clear flare-up the next day, giving pain and stiffness in my back, neck, front of chest, and side of the rib cage. This wasn't the first time I felt pain in my ribcage; sometimes a sharp tightness would appear in the front centre of my chest, felt with deep breathing, but relieved with stretching. I was concerned more about the advancement of pain in my torso, but my rheumatologist was more concerned with the inflammation in my foot at that time, since the fluid present during swelling is the fluid that causes permanent damage to the joint. In 2021, I received a follow-up x-ray of my back, and the sclerosis in my SI joint had not progressed. This inspired me to continue with my efforts to this day.

## Personal symptoms that may have been preliminary signs of AS

My main bout of arthritis and diagnosis of the condition didn't occur until I was 36. However, once I started investigating the condition, I realized that I had many health issues earlier in life that may have been preliminary signals of the condition. They included many foot problems, including bursitis in my feet, fallen arches at around age 17, and Achilles tendonitis at age 20, for which I received cortisone shots. This was preceded by gastrointestinal illness, and trauma to my foot during athletics training. In retrospect, this was perhaps the clearest early signal that I might develop AS later in life (hindsight being 20/20 of course). The heel and Achilles pain that returned during my main bout of arthritis were the same.

At age 17, I also developed a TMJ disorder. During my thirties, this area was quiet, but after my AS onset it became an ongoing issue; painful with clicking and locking. AS can potentially affect any joint, however, non-inflammatory TMJ disorders are common, and that was more likely in my particular case.

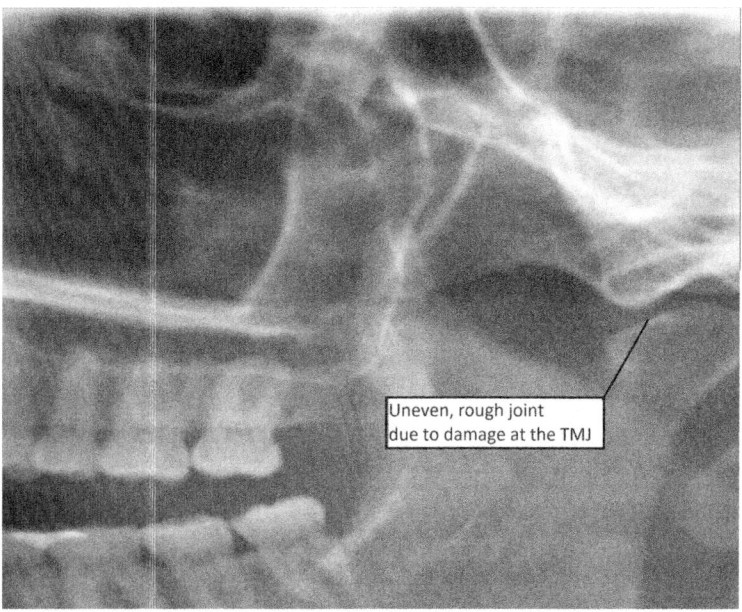

While AS predominately affects the back, I didn't suffer in that area until lower-back pain began to develop, in the SI joint region at age 35. I remember blaming this on holding awkward postures while carrying my third child as a baby.

Gut problems were persistent throughout my life, and I can clearly recall major and frequent gastrointestinal infections, most often when travelling overseas, at ages 25, 27, 30 and 33, involving diarrhea and fever, and I was often prescribed antibiotics.

Age 36, the beginning of my major bout of AS symptoms started with a return trip from overseas in 2016, when I had to sleep on a cot in the terminal for a cancelled flight. This is when I first noticed gastrointestinal illness and the beginning of my major bout of AS symptoms. My initial symptoms in July 2016 (chills, back pain, high fever, vomiting, nausea) were consistent with a *Klebsiella* infection.

After these initial digestive and fever-like symptoms, the first joint pain occurred in my big toe.

> *"Infection usually settles in a single joint, at least at first. The pain from the infection is different and much worse than the usual pain of OA or RA. It keeps you awake at night, and brings tears when the joint is moved. Fever or chills may be clues to the true nature of the problem, but may not appear at first." "Arthritis, Thompson, P.225"*

In retrospect, I seemed to be having a classic onset of arthritis. From this point on, I started receiving a number of tests and diagnoses that all began to paint a clear picture of an ankylosing spondylitis diagnosis, including testing positive for the HLA-B27 marker, having elevated C-reactive protein during blood tests (42 mg/L at highest point), good response to NSAIDS, and dactylitis, sacroiliitis, and plantar fasciitis all in 2016. Furthermore, I tested positive for mononucleosis in 2016. Interestingly, this test has been noted at times to be a false positive for *Klebsiella*. (Ridker PM, 1990)

## Tracking inflammation and blood markers

When I was first diagnosed with AS, I went for regular blood tests to track inflammation levels and other markers in my blood that provided a window into my condition. With this data, was able to track markers like liver enzymes and C-reactive protein to understand my progress. With my daily log, I was then able to overlap my blood tests with changes in diet, medication, and activity, and to look for correlations and causes. I also paid attention to the level of pain along the way, as it often acted as a clue to the cause of my condition.

*Enzymes in the blood*

Every two months, I was required to go for a blood test to check for a host of inflammation markers.

Tests on the standing order card were:

- ALT - Alanine transaminase is the enzyme released by the liver when it is damaged or diseased. This test checks for liver disease, especially cirrhosis, hepatitis, damage caused by medications, alcohol, or viruses.
- ANA - Antinuclear antibodies that play a role in rheumatic disease.
- AST - Aspartate aminotransferases is a liver enzyme, similar to ALT.
- CREA – Creatine, to check for kidney function.
- CRP - C-reactive protein to measure inflammation.
- Hb - Hemoglobin to check for anemia.
- Neutrophils and lymphocytes (white blood cells used to fight off an infection), as a low count can be caused by autoimmune disorders.

# MY PERSONAL EXPERIENCE WITH AS

## A typical blood test result would look like this:

| | Flags Results | Reference Range | Units |
|---|---|---|---|
| **Hematology** | | | |
| WBC | 4.5 | 4.0-10.0 | 10*9/L |
| RBC | 4.68 | 4.20-5.40 | 10*12/L |
| Hemoglobin | 143 | 135-170 | g/L |
| Hematocrit | 0.43 | 0.40-0.50 | L/L |
| MCV | 91 | 82-98 | fl |
| MCH | 30.6 | 27.5-33.5 | pg |
| MCHC | 335 | 300-370 | g/L |
| RDW | 13.9 | 11.5-14.5 | % |
| Platelet Count | 191 | 150-400 | 10*9/L |
| **Differential** | | | |
| Neutrophils | 2.2 | 2.0-7.5 | 10*9/L |
| Lymphocytes | 1.8 | 1.0-4.0 | 10*9/L |
| Monocytes | 0.4 | 0.1-0.8 | 10*9/L |
| Eosinophils | 0 | 0.0-0.7 | 10*9/L |
| Basophils | 0 | 0.0-0.2 | 10*9/L |
| Granulocytes Immature | 0 | 0.0-0.1 | 10*9/L |
| **General Chemistry** | | | |
| Creatinine | 76 | 45-110 | umol/L |
| Estimated GFR | 110 | >=60 | |
| | Units for eGFR are mL/min/1.73sq.m Kidney function estimate based on assumption of a stable serum creatinine concentration: diet, drugs, pregnancy, clinical state and muscle mass can affect accuracy of the estimate. Urinary ACR may assist interpretation. See www.bcguidelines.ca/pdf/ckd.pdf | | |
| ALT | 25 | <50 | U/L |
| AST | 18 | <36 | U/L |
| **Serum Proteins** | | | |
| C Reactive Protein (High Sensitivity) | 0.3 | <4.8 | mg/L |
| | New reference range effective 09/11/2017. | | |
| | Interpretation: This high sensitivity CRP method is sensitive to 0.3 mg/L and is suitable for coronary artery disease assessment and detection of active inflammation. | | |
| **Immunology** | | | |
| Nuclear Ab Titre | Neg | Titre <1:80 | |
| | HEp-2000 cell substrate for indirect | | |

immunofluorescence shows improved sensitivity for SS-A/Ro antibodies.

Negative: Antinuclear antibodies (ANAs) are commonly detected in the sera of patients with systemic autoimmune rheumatic diseases (SARD). Specimen was screened at 1:80 titre. A negative test rarely needs to be repeated unless there is a strong clinical suspicion of evolving disease or a clinical change suggesting diagnostic review.

## *C-reactive protein*

C-reactive protein (CRP) is a substance produced by the liver that increases in the presence of inflammation in the body. An elevated CRP level is identified with blood tests and is considered a non-specific "marker" for disease. It can signal flare-ups of inflammatory diseases such AS.

During the course of my symptoms, I was scheduled for regular blood tests. The following is a log of my CRP levels, recorded on a regular basis over a period of about four years:

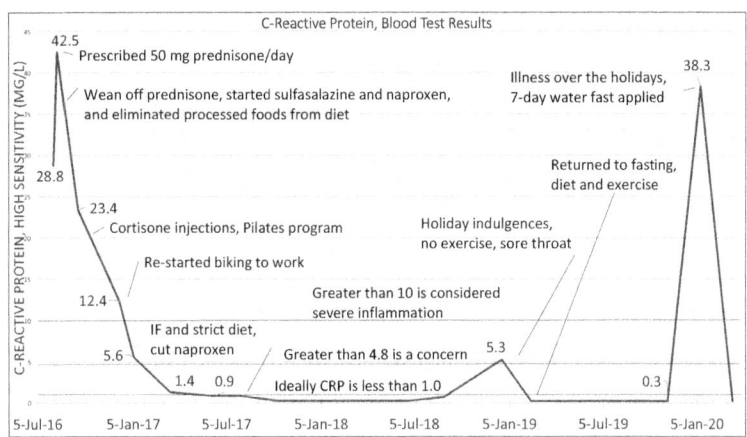

*CRP Chart. This chart documents my CRP levels, based on blood test results from the onset of severe symptoms in 2016, to my condition in March 2020, with notes to offer suggestions of correlations to spikes in CRP levels. The Y-axis reports high sensitivity CRP levels in mg/L.*

Greater than 10 mg/L is considered severe inflammation, 4.8 is cause for concern, 2 is high risk, and ideally the reading should be less than 1, although different labs use different cut-offs for this measure.

Initially, medications greatly helped to reduce my CRP and get me back into exercising, and they provided me with a chance to change my diet. Very noteworthy, is the spike of 38.3 mg/L in early 2020. In January 2020, I again fell sick with IBD, fever, fatigue, chills and back pain, like the onset in 2016. I applied seven days of water fasting. My CRP on day six of my fast was 38.3 mg/L, and since then was sharply reduced. This correlated closely to my BASDAI. I was able to stay active, and pain subsided without medication after seven days. I have been able to apply this technic to suppress flare-ups, in combination with diet, exercise, stretching, and stress management, staying medication free.

There are many causes and strategies to consider when addressing elevated CRP levels. Most importantly, in addition to fasting, exercise and an anti-inflammatory diet are a means to reduce CRP levels:

> *"Dr. Weil recommends an anti-inflammatory diet that includes two to three servings of fish such as salmon or sardines per week. If you don't eat fish, he suggests taking fish oil supplements. He also recommends taking anti-inflammatory herbs including ginger and turmeric and following your doctor's recommendations for heart health. That means quitting smoking, watching your diet (particularly avoid foods that predominantly consist of flour and/or sugar), and getting regular exercise: research indicates that as fitness levels decline, C-reactive protein levels go up." (Weil, 2018) (C-Reactive Protein Test, 2018) (Solutions, 2018) (WebMD, 2018)*

# CHAPTER 3

## MEDICAL TREATMENTS

I've found a number of treatments that have been effective for me in managing ankylosing spondylitis. There is medicine, which helped me greatly during the height of my symptoms, but of course it has side effects and can cause long-term damage to the body. Diet, fasting, exercise and a positive mindset (knowing that you *can* get better) are definitely the way to go, especially once your symptoms are reasonably under control and you are at the point where you need to develop a long-term management plan, since AS is a life-long condition. The more I researched the medications I was taking, the more I learned of their benefits, but also of their risks.

Over the course of my treatment, I was prescribed a number of drugs, some more effective than others. Initially, I received celecoxib (200 mg), and cyclobenzaprine (10 mg), a muscle relaxant. I didn't seem to notice any benefit from the celecoxib, and the cyclobenzaprine caused significant drowsiness to the point that I couldn't function with it. I received antibiotics, prednisone, local cortisone injections, sulfasalazine, and naproxen. Per my rheumatologist, I was prescribed naproxen to treat my back and sulfasalazine to treat peripheral arthritis in the feet and hands and knee. For more information on effectiveness, see "What worked, what didn't" in chapter 10.

There are a few of main methods used to medically treat AS.

## TNFα suppression

TNFα (tumor necrosis factor, alpha) is a natural protein in the body that is involved in inflammation. It acts as a signalling component in the body's immune system that is used when infection or tissue injury occurs. Anti-TNFα drugs (or TNF antagonists) are drugs that suppress the TNFα, which is a main medical approach for managing AS. Several studies have shown that TNFα blocking agents, such as infliximab, etanercept, and adalimumab are highly effective in reducing inflammation and reducing the disease activity in arthritis patients. These are all considered disease-modifying anti-rheumatic drugs (DMARDs), and are typically expensive, required to be delivered by injection, and are often effective, but typically a second line of attack, if the less-expensive and more commonly available NSAIDs are not effective.

Another reason to suppress TNFα in AS patients is to control bone formation, and hopefully prevent the fusing of the bones in the spine. One study showed that three years of TNFα-blocking therapy resulted in a significant increase of bone formation after three months, and the process continued at a higher level for up to three years. The study suggests that reducing TNFα levels can improve bone mineral density and formation in a positive way, by suppressing the inflammatory aspect of AS. (José Francisco Zambrano-Zaragoza, US National Library of Medicine National Institutes of Health, 2013) Before this study, it was believed that NSAIDs were the only drug able to assist with bone formation, through the same mechanism of reducing inflammation.

(Ippokratis Pountos, 2012) There are some downsides to suppressing TNFα to a high extent. More recent studies in 2017 showed that anti-TNF therapy and the reactivation of latent tuberculosis (TB) can occur. (Fabrizio Cantini, 2017)

Interestingly, by researching diet, I've come to learn that some of the most effective foods that you can add to your diet to manage AS also suppress TNFα, and therefore suppress inflammation through a similar mechanism as these medications. Therefore, I would strongly recommend including any foods that suppress TNFα in your diet, as they are the mainstay of medical treatment. More on this later.

## COX-1/COX-2 suppression

Cyclooxygenase 1 and 2 (COX-1 and COX-2) are naturally occurring enzymes involved in generating inflammation in the body. They are involved in the metabolism of arachidonic acid (AA) (a type of omega-6 fat) into prostaglandins that are involved in inflammation. NSAIDs, like naproxen or indomethacin, suppress COX-1 and COX-2.

Naproxen is non-selective in suppressing both COX-1 and COX-2, while some NSAIDs, like celecoxib, focus on suppressing COX-2. This medication was designed to focus on only the inflammation involved in arthritis, while not causing damage to the gastrointestinal system such as gastrointestinal bleeding, which is associated with COX-1 suppression. However, it created other side effects instead, like in the cases of rofecoxib and valdecoxib, which were both withdrawn from the market because of heat attack and stroke risks. Celecoxib is still available and generally effective, but it has its own list of gastrointestinal side effects like diarrhea and flatulence, and more severe side effects like kidney or heart failure. Furthermore, the strategy to focus on COX-2 suppression does not seem to alleviate damage to the gastrointestinal system, since it has since been discovered that COX-1 and COX-2 are both necessary for stomach lining maintenance and vascular tone (F HALTER, 2001)

Some foods have been found to suppress COX-1 and COX-2 and suppress prostaglandins, without these side effects. And of course, the diet can be changed to reduce the omega-6 oils consumed, again, without side effects.

## NSAIDs

> "One dangerous paradox in arthritis treatment is that the drugs most commonly used to treat arthritis are toxins to this intestinal barrier. All commonly used nonsteroidal anti-inflammatory drugs (like [ibuprofen], etc.), apart from aspirin and nabumetone, are associated with increased intestinal permeability in man. While reversible in the short term, it may take months to improve the barrier following prolonged use." (Baillieres Clin Rheumatol 10:165, 1996).

Naproxen is not without its risks and side effects too. When I was prescribed naproxen, I was also prescribed a proton pump inhibitor to reduce stomach acid and protect the stomach from damage while taking the naproxen. It should be noted here that proton pump inhibitors, a class of medication that are used to reduce stomach acid, are associated with an increased risk of developing small intestinal bacterial overgrowth (SIBO). SIBO is also associated with rosacea, which I developed for the first time in my life after several months taking these medications.

Naproxen works by temporarily blocking the body's production of prostaglandins, which play a direct role in pain and inflammation (it is a prostaglandin antagonist). It is a non-selective COX inhibitor, compared to celecoxib, which is a selective COX-2 inhibitor. Furthermore, while studies showed that naproxen was found to promote collagen synthesis, it unfortunately inhibited proper enthesis repair.

Prostaglandin cell receptors include DP1-2, EP1-4, FP, IP1-2, and TP, which function for (among other things) regulating inflammation, regulating calcium movement, acting on the thermoregulatory centre of hypothalamus to produce fever, and acting on parietal cells in the stomach wall to inhibit acid secretion.

NSAIDs influence the AA pathway to inflammation (O'Connor, 2013). These functions, regulated by prostaglandins, are not bad in the correct intensity and duration. In fact, studies show that COX-2 activity is also important in resolving inflammation, so we don't want to turn off its function completely or for too long. This may be the most important side effect of naproxen in relation to AS, since this process, when taking naproxen for a long duration, may actually lead to chronic inflammatory conditions. (Thomas A Perry, 2021)

Instead of taking NSAIDs like naproxen, indomethacin or celecoxib, I took the strategy of reducing my body's inflammatory activity by reducing my consumption of AA– and linoleic acid (LA)–containing foods. With a natural and healthy diet, my focus was to obtain a balance between omega-6 and omega-3 oils to reduce the inflammatory oils, but also permit the healing functions of COX-1 and COX-2. At the same time, I was fortunately able to wean myself from NSAIDS.

## DMARDs

Disease-modifying anti-rheumatic drugs (DMARDs) are immunosuppressive agents and can be conventional or a genetically engineered (biologic) form. They are a more targeted therapy, typically for inflammatory arthritis, but also used for connective tissue disease or even some types of cancers. They are also not without their own side effects.

## Sulfasalazine

Sulfasalazine (SSZ) is classified as a DMARD, and it is generally regarded as a frontline medication, taken orally. Importantly in AS, sulfasalazine suppresses the HLA-B27 gene (Hui-Chun Yu, 2016), which has a close association to the disease. Generally, there are mixed reviews as to its efficacy, with one study concluding *"that there is no evidence for a clinically relevant benefit on spinal symptoms or function, but sulfasalazine may have a role in peripheral joint disease associated with spondyloarthritis"* (J Zochling, 2005). Another source also referrers to mixed efficacy: *"North American experience with this drug in the treatment of RA has been limited, but since it's a mainstay in the treatment of inflammatory bowel disease, its side effects are well known. The British seem to be quite enthusiastic, and to rank it somewhere near intramuscular gold. Its safety profile is very encouraging, it's fairly effective, and it takes action in two to three months. Its benefits are sustained moderately well over the long term. There are conflicting reports as to whether sulfasalazine is useful in some of the seronegative arthritis conditions, particularly psoriatic arthritis and AS."* Arthritis, Thompson, P251.

Interestingly, sulfasalazine is compared to being no more effective than placebo, *"SSZ [sulfasalazine] was no better than placebo for the treatment of the signs and symptoms of uSpA [undifferentiated Spondyloarthrapies]; however, SSZ was more effective than placebo in the subgroup of patients with IBP and no peripheral arthritis."* (J Braun, 2006). This last study I found surprising, as my rheumatologist specifically prescribed me sulfasalazine for peripheral arthritis, and I have read in other sources that it is intended for peripheral arthritis and not the spine. During the height of my symptoms, I was personally treated with SSZ for a period of 12 months. I would agree, based on my own observations, that it is not the most effective for the spine, particularly the neck, as my neck pain first developed even while I was on a full dosage of sulfasalazine. This is a slow-acting medication, taking four weeks to reach full dosage, and when I discontinued the drug, I felt no change until three-and-a-half months later, when I started to log a marked increase in foot arthritis flare-ups and overnight stiffness. This approximately three-month delay in a return of symptoms was, impressively, predicted by my rheumatologist.

Another interesting benefit from sulfasalazine, is its benefit for the gut, which seemed serendipitous in the case of AS, as I believe it addresses the other area of the body that seems to be suffering from inflammation. It has been shown to provide immunosuppressive effects on intestinal immune responses, and it has been proposed that sulfasalazine can diminish intestinal mucosal permeability. So, while it's reducing joint inflammation, it may, at the same time, be preventing interaction between *Klebsiella* in the gut, the HLA-B27 gene, and the immune response. This response was also noticed to be distinctly beneficial in AS, as opposed to controls in patients with RA. (M Hvatum†, The gut–joint axis: cross reactive food antibodies in rheumatoid arthritis, 2006). Coincidently, I received sulfasalazine from my rheumatologist, which I was able to take orally, and which may have ended up being an effective choice since there was evidence it could also treat my bowel problems.

Another interesting, beneficial side effect of sulfasalazine is its effect on the *Klebsiella* bacteria, which I will discuss in more detail as a suspected cause of AS: *"A significant decrease in the concentration of Klebsiella pneumoniae IgA antibodies for 26 weeks treatment with sulfasalazine has been reported in Finnish AS patients when compared to controls (Nissila et al. 1994). It would appear that the antimicrobial component in sulfasalazine is sulfapyridine (Taggart et al. 1996) and could be acting against the bowel microbial flora."* (A. Ebringer, 1996) (Ebringer A., Ankylosing Spondylitis and Klebsiella, 2012). I personally feel that sulfasalazine provided me with much benefit during the year I was using it. Side effects include rash and sun sensitivity, decreased sperm counts, and a requirement to check liver and blood counts every one to three months to monitor for other adverse effects.

## Methotrexate

My rheumatologist discussed other therapies with me, including the trial use of biologics such as infliximab and adalimumab. However, I feared the idea of having to inject myself with medication on a regular basis to get through my days, so it helped motivate me toward natural solutions. Like sulfasalazine, methotrexate also requires liver and blood tests for monitoring. Methotrexate, along with intramuscular gold have both been found to be effective in the use of psoriatic arthritis but their use is limited by their toxicity. Gold is no longer used.

## Hydroxychloroquine

Hydroxychloroquine is another DMARD that has been shown to reduce the pain and swelling of arthritis. Originally used to treat malaria, it's now prescribed for diagnoses like RA, lupus, juvenile idiopathic arthritis or other autoimmune conditions. Typically, it's taken by oral tablet and also has a delay of several months before benefits can be noticed. It's generally considered well tolerated, but long-term use can cause damage to the eyes, and so regular eye checks to monitor for drug toxicity are recommended after five years of use.

## Biologics

Biologics, or biosimilars, are a special class of genetically engineered DMARDs that are made from biological sources and highly focused to modify a specific function of the immune system pathway. Some examples include certolizumab, secukinumab, etanercept, adalimumab, infliximab and golimumab, most of which target TNFα, or cytokines such as IL-17, IL-12 or IL-23. * (Hoffman-La Roche, Enbrel Canada Inc, AbbVie Corporation, Bristol-Myers Squibb Canada, Janssen Inc, Pfizer Canada Inc., 2015, 2016).

Often, a combination of two or three DMARDs can be tried for better efficacy. I was fortunate enough to be able to get my symptoms under control before having to resort to biologics. Since my personal experience with these medications is very limited, I can't comment on their effectiveness from a firsthand perspective.

## Steroids

### Prednisone

Prednisone is a powerful, steroidal anti-inflammatory. It's often used as a front line defence and is effective as a firefighting measure when symptoms are severe, but its side effects can be significant. Consider this assessment by John Thompson, MD:

> *When corticosteroids are used in doses of more than the equivalent of 7.5 mg of prednisone a day, the adrenal gland does not make cortisol. This is not a problem if drugs like prednisone are used for short periods only. But when such doses are used continuously for prolonged periods (three months is considered the cut-off), cortisol production will be completely suppressed. The patient is*

*now dependent on a source outside the body for corticosteroid. Since corticosteroids are essential for life and are particularly important in helping the body deal with major physical stress, their sudden absence - if for any reason the patient stops taking daily prednisone - can have serious consequences. If adrenal gland suppression is only partial, symptoms of fatigue, nausea, loss of appetite and muscle pain may develop. If suppression is total, the patient may experience the life-threatening state doctors call 'shock'. The only safe way to reduce, and stop, corticosteroids is slowly, over a period of weeks to months. But even if the patient has managed to achieve this, the body may not completely recover its ability to produce large amounts of cortisol in circumstances of stress until a year or more goes by (J. Thompson, 1996).*

This 7.5 mg/day level really puts things into perspective for me, when I look back at my notes and see that I was prescribed 25 mg/day, and later 50 mg/day, for my initial symptoms. Rheumatologists typically do not use such a high dose; however, this is sometimes used by gastroenterologists for treatment of IBD. This was obviously a hard and fast firefighting measure to stop the inflammation cascade, and it seemed to have helped, but it was not a long-term solution. I suffered some significant side effects in a short time frame (13 days) from prednisone, the most worrisome being heart palpitations; I felt I needed to call my doctor to request a reduction in dosage. After only 19 days of using the medication, I was instructed by my doctor to slowly wean myself off it over the next 30 days, and most symptoms cleared shortly after, although intermittent heart palpitations continued for a good five or six months afterwards.

## Cortisone injections

Cortisone injections are also a steroid, containing synthetic cortisol that is injected locally at a joint to reduce local inflammation. They are also very effective, but they can eventually cause damage to the cartilage at a joint, and the number of times they can be used is limited. There are even reports that they become less effective the more they are administered. I feel like I've received more cortisone injections than any one person should receive. My first injections were well before I was diagnosed with AS. In my early twenties, I suffered from Achilles tendonitis and plantar fasciitis pain that extended right into my big toe. I had X-rays and an MRI scan, but no damage or injury was clear. I wore a brace for six months to immobilize the joint to allow it to heal, but to no avail. My doctor at the time was not able to provide me with a diagnosis but was confident the cortisone injections in the heel would resolve the issue. I found it to be a very painful injection, but after a few days, the pain cleared. After limping on it for six months, I was happy to be back to my active self again.

After being diagnosed with AS, at age 36, I received several cortisone injections to relieve peripheral arthritis. The arthritis symptoms in my feet were identical to those I remember from my twenties, so I wonder if it was an early sign of a pending AS condition later in life. In total, I received four shots in the second toe of my left foot, one shot in the largest knuckle of my left-hand index finger, and two shots in the second toe of my righthand foot. In all cases, the shots provided immediate local relief the next day and continued relief in the long term. In most cases, it was an immediate relief in swelling, followed by a more gradual relief in pain and increase in movement over the next several days after the injection. Once I was off other medications and about two years into the disease in July 2018, I received one last cortisone shot in my righthand second toe, where I had synovitis and ongoing swelling that I couldn't relieve through icing, rest or other means. The swelling immediately went down, but this time the shot didn't resolve the pain or sensitivity to pressure while walking. My mobility improved, and pain was lessened, but it persisted, and the foot was sensitive to pressure. A general RICE (Rest, Ice, Compression, Elevation) strategy was effective in bringing down the remaining inflammation and pain in this location in my foot. Taking a three-week break from cycling was the final step I needed to resolve the issue where I received the cortisone shot. This last shot seemed the least effective out of all shots I received. This area of pain also seemed to be more related to repetitive use injury than arthritis. Initially, pain increased with rest (I believe this was the arthritis side of things talking), but after about two weeks the pain and swelling cleared. Finally, fixing shoe problems (with flat shoes and a bigger toe box) and avoiding overuse ended up being the longer-term solution that seemed to allow the joint to heal over the following month.

From all these injections, the only case that I felt any side effects from was the injection in my index finger. The first was a burst blood vessel at the location of the injection, causing significant internal bruising and swelling. I had broken a blood vessel here before, so I'm not convinced it was caused by the injection, but I wonder if the injection increased susceptibility to future injury. This injury occurred a long nine months after the injection. The second, only a month after the broken blood vessel, was numbness/tingling in the finger. This symptom occurred in other fingers as well, so again, I can't be sure this was caused by the injection.

## Supplements

Supplements can also run the risk of causing side effects, due to the possibility of taking them in doses much higher than available in nature. For example, studies show that antioxidants can lessen symptoms of AS and arthritis in general, however, too much vitamin C may cause other complications such as kidney stones. While I did take many supplements to try to treat my condition, I treated this as a transitional strategy; my end goal was to replace supplements with diet in the long term. I've replaced vitamin C tablets with whole foods containing enough quantities of vitamin C. However, I still do rely on some supplements, such as DHA and EPA omega-3 oils, which I personally find very beneficial and safe when taken regularly and over a long enough time frame. See my recommended foods section for more detail on supplements.

## Topical treatments

### Essential oils

I also tested some topical treatments for my peripheral arthritis. I used a spray containing all-natural active ingredients, using menthol, eucalyptus oil and clove oil, each having evidence of efficacy.

Menthol, applied as a topical agent, counteracts irritation through a cooling effect and by stimulating nociceptors and then desensitizing them. Topically applied menthol may also activate central analgesic pathways. (Pergolizzi JV Jr1 & Group., 2018)

Essential oils of *Eucalyptus citriodora* (EC), *Eucalyptus tereticornis* (ET) and *Eucalyptus globulus* (EG) induced analgesic effects in two models of testing, both peripherally and centrally acting, and they also produced anti-inflammatory effects. (Silva J1, 2003)

When tested against placebos, both clove oil and benzocaine gels had significantly lower mean pain scores. Both clove and benzocaine were considered equally effective. (Silva J1, 2003) (Alqareer A1, 2006)

In my personal experience with these essential oils, I apply them to the top of the ball of the foot, below, and on heel. They provide a strong cooling effect on the foot, especially on top. They do not fully relive joint pain, but they do provide good relief through cooling. Benefit at the heel is similar but less pronounced. On my lower back, they also provide good cooling relief. A topical treatment like this is exactly what it says it is, topical. It only affects the surface; it doesn't provide deep penetrating pain relief into the joint. At best it will last a few hours.

## Diclofenac

Diclofenac is an NSAID, much like naproxen, but is applied topically for local relief. Being locally applied, in my experience, it has a much deeper and longer-lasting effect. However, side effects are the same as naproxen. The essential oils had a relatively immediate but short-term effect. Conversely, the diclofenac (like naproxen) was most effective over a longer period, when re-applied as prescribed over a period of four or more days.

## Vagal nerve stimulation

A vagal nerve stimulator (VNS) is in the category of electroceuticals—electrical devices that provide health benefit by using electrical impulses like a pacemaker. A VNS is a device that is implanted in the neck, with wires that wrap around one branch of the vagus nerve and deliver mild electrical impulses at pre-set intervals. It has very recently been given FDA approval for use for managing migraines and has other applications such as managing epilepsy and depression. It is now being trialled to manage autoimmune conditions such as RA, Crohn's disease, and lupus; AS would fit in this category as well. The concept for autoimmune conditions is new, and there are significant potential side effects that include cardiac arrest and bradycardia, but at the same time, this therapy shows promise for these serious conditions by focusing on a specific nerve, as opposed to drugs that travel through the body and affect other tissues and have side effects of their own. Interestingly, the vagus nerve is the most important connection between the gut and brain, and this seems to fit the overall theory of gut involvement in arthritis. VNS is something we may hear more of in the future if these initial trials are successful.

## Drug financial conflicts

I never had any interest in taking drugs to deal with AS for the long term. In fact, getting off medications so I could be healthy for the sake of my family, was one of my biggest driving motivators. I was already strongly motivated to avoid medications. I also wasn't ignorant of the financial motivations of the pharmaceutical industry, which ideally should be putting patients before profits. However, it hit particularly close to home when I found an article discussing how cleverly and carefully FDA advisors receive financial benefits from pharmaceutical companies. (Charles Piller, 2018)

Adalimumab and etanercept were medications that were offered to me to control AS—they were highlighted as expensive but effective options—if we showed that more common DMARDs like sulfasalazine and methotrexate were not effective. I felt some pressure to move on to the next, more powerful medication, but in the back of my mind, I wasn't going to push through DMARDs so I could switch over to biologics as soon as possible. I was personally trying to de-escalate the drug war going on inside my body. I was doing everything I could to get off sulfasalazine and I was afraid to even get myself going on methotrexate. Then I read about tofacitinib, which was a methotrexate substitute currently in use for RA, and currently (at the time of writing this book) in studies for its effectiveness in AS.

Tofacitinib, was approved by the FDA but not approved by European regulatory agencies because of concerns of efficacy and safety. Then how did this drug get approved by the FDA? This same article notes that during the approval of this drug, FDA advisors received significant funds from drug manufacturers. Advisors are supposed to declare conflicts of interests, which would include payments from pharmaceutical companies. However, they don't receive payment during their advisory role—they receive payment afterward, after the drug has been approved—which makes these payments that much more difficult to track. As of 2016, tofacitinib was undergoing a phase II trial for ankylosing spondylitis.

As an update in November 2020, in phase III testing of the drug tofacitinib, "patients with ankylosing spondylitis demonstrated rapid clinical response to tofacitinib, which produced significantly greater efficacy than placebo, but with more adverse events," according to the study's lead investigator, Atul Deodhar, MD, professor of medicine at Oregon Health & Science University in Portland. While it's good to hear positive results on efficacy, it appears that safety is still a concern.

There are many effective medications out there, and they've helped me on my own road to recovery, but from my own experience, most come with side effects. As a patient, you can become dependent on them for pain and inflammation relief, instead of making the difficult but important lifestyle and diet changes to avoid inflammation naturally. By suppressing symptoms, they hide deeper causes of your health issues, such as food sensitivities and lack of exercise. Be an advocate for your own health. Work with your health professionals to take what you need, develop a plan to get off medications, and don't give up.

# CHAPTER 4

# CAUSES

I had some symptoms in my youth that might have indicated arthritis was coming, if I had known what to look for. I even had a year of escalating back pain before my major onset, but in my situation, I had a very clear "beginning" to my AS. It was like someone flipped a switch, and things never returned to normal. One week I was functioning as I always had, the next I was in a downward spiral and physically very limited. A clear start like this suggested a trigger; it suggested causes. I could not help but try to investigate. Was it caused by allergies, bacteria, viruses, or genes? What made it worse and what made it better?

## Free radicals

You've most likely heard of the dangers of free radicals roaming our bodies and causing damage and ill health. But what are free radicals? What's happening in the body, and what can we do to prevent it? Being an engineer, I like to think of the mechanical equivalent, and in this case it's quite similar to the rust we see occurring on a car or on a boat. The water (especially salty water, when road salt combines with moisture) can be paralleled with a free radical that causes the oxidative damage in the body, much like rust on the metal body of your car. In the body, it is the reactive oxygen species (ROS) that carries an unpaired electron (hydroxide ion) that reacts with the chemistry that makes up our cells. This is caused by exposure to radiation, pollution, excessive exercise, emotional or physical stress, and even oxygen itself, but also foods including sugar and sweeteners, additives, certain medications, and unhealthy fats like the oxidized fats that are often found in processed and refined foods. It's something we can't get entirely away from because it's also a by-product of a normal, healthy metabolism. However, instead of causing rust in the body, ROS in the body causes disease, and there is evidence it contributes to autoimmune disease.

The hydroxide ion is generated in substantial amounts in chronic inflammatory conditions due to increased oxidative stress. Inflammation itself creates free radicals, causing cellular damage and cellular death, also known as apoptosis. This is a negative feedback loop that contributes to increased inflammation in the body.

> *"Reactive oxygen species play a role in apoptosis. NF-kB, which is a collective term to describe the Rel family of transcription factors, inhibits apoptosis by upregulating several antiapoptotic genes [17]. Conversely, the c-Jun N-terminal kinase (JNK) promotes apoptosis when activated for prolonged periods [20]. Prolonged activation has been shown to be caused by exposure to ROS directly as well as by inactivating JNK inhibitors such as MAP Kinase phosphatases [20]. Suppression of TNFα-induced ROS accumulation seems to be the mechanism by which NF-kB downregulates JNK activation."* (H Ahsan, 2003)

In other words, prolonged exposure to free radicals causes cell damage, but it also can suppress cell death, resulting in a lot of damaged cells hanging around.

## Solutions to free radicals - antioxidants

A car can be made from steel so that it doesn't rust, or it is coated to prevent exposure to water and salt. Relating this to our bodies, we can reduce our exposure to smoke or synthetic chemicals, but some ROS, like hydrogen peroxide, which is a harmful by-product of many normal metabolic processes, comes from within and cannot simply be avoided. Antioxidants come into play here. In this scenario, a catalyst enzyme helps the hydrogen peroxide convert into water and oxygen before the hydrogen peroxide has a chance to do much damage.

## Preventive antioxidants - glutathione

Glutathione breaks down hydrogen peroxide in a unique fashion and is recognized as being possibly the most important intra-cellular defence against damage from ROS. Our bodies can produce their own glutathione if we provide the building blocks required for them to do so.

How? Increase your body's ability to produce glutathione. Sulfur is required for the body to synthesize glutathione. Eat sulfur-rich foods containing methionine and cysteine like beef, fish and poultry proteins; vegetables like broccoli, Brussels sprouts, cauliflower, kale, watercress and mustard greens; and also, allium vegetables, like garlic shallots, and onions. Eat foods high in selenium like beef, chicken, fish, and organ meats.

## Isoflavones

Isoflavones comprise a subclass of the naturally occurring plant substance group called phenolic flavonoids, and they have a structure similar to estrogen. Isoflavones are produced almost exclusively by the members of the Fabaceae (i.e., Leguminosae, or bean) family. Soybeans, which contain high amounts of the isoflavone genistein, are a common source of isoflavones in human food. Genistein can act as a phytoestrogen in mammals. Although phytoestrogens are not steroids, they can alter activity of the estrogen receptor. Some isoflavones are termed antioxidants because of their ability to trap singlet oxygen. Genistein has been shown to suppress the inflammatory activity of NF-kB when inflammatory AA fatty acids are included in the diet. It also supports the anti-inflammatory activity of dietary DHA fatty acid against breast cancer.

## Flavanols

The subclass flavanols are the most common of flavonoids in food. The flavonoid quercetin has been shown to have anticancer activity by multiple mechanisms including induction of apoptosis (a cellular "cleaning" mechanism) and inhibition of COX-2 activity. As mentioned earlier, inhibiting COX-2 is a strategy of some medications. Quercetin has also been shown to inhibit NF-kB, also a strategy of some medications in an effort to reduce inflammation.

## Hydroxycinnamic acids

Hydroxycinnamic acids naturally occur in various foods and inhibit the NF-kB in the body that contributes to inflammation. They have been shown to have benefit against multiple diseases, at least partly by protecting against oxidative stress and inflammatory damage. They are found in foods such as artichokes, apples, strawberries and blueberries and coffee, and herbs and spices such as basil, thyme, oregano, echinacea and aloe. Polyphenols in general are micronutrients packed with antioxidants that can help reduce inflammation in all autoimmune diseases. (Reiko Nagasaka 1, 2007)

*Scavenging antioxidants—vitamin C*

On boats, often we use zincs for protection from rust. They are a sacrificial zinc anode on a boat that allows the zinc to react more readily with the ions in the water. The zinc will rust first, protecting the hull of the boat in the process. This is similar to the activity of scavenging antioxidants in the body. If we eat the right foods, we can introduce antioxidants into our bodies that will react with free radicals, such as hydrogen peroxide, before they cause damage in the body and protect our cells in the process. Probably, the best example of an antioxidant acting this way is melatonin, which is considered "suicidal" and is sacrificed in the oxidation-reduction reaction with a free radical. Other scavenging antioxidants include vitamin E and beta carotene (vitamin A).

Another AS patient I interviewed found significant relief by using copious amounts of vitamin C supplements, on the order of 10,000 mg per day. While his testimony does support the theory that free radicals contribute to AS and antioxidants are part of the solution, I cannot recommend such high quantities of vitamin C. While the body has the means of removing too much vitamin C, high amounts can increase the risk of developing kidney stones, particularly in men (Pietro Manuel Ferraro, 2015). Obtaining vitamin C from diet is a much safer method. In following up with this individual, I was happy to hear that he had abandoned his strategy of vitamin C megadoses and is managing through more natural strategies.

*The final step in the strategy—fasting*

Remember all the cell damage, but lack of programmed cell death, to clear out old cells? This is where fasting plays its part. Fasting will not only reduce exposure to free radicals, upregulating programmed cell death, but also increase autophagy, the self-consumption of defective or damaged parts of cells. More on fasting later.

## Pro-Inflammatory Cytokines

Cytokines, like IL-17 and IL-23, are proteins involved in cell signalling that can cause inflammation.

> *"Based on preclinical models and human GWAS studies and pharmacogenomic disease association analyses, psoriasis, IBD, and AS have emerged as the leading disease indications for anti-IL-17 and anti-IL-23."* (Sarah L. Gaffen, 2015)

There are a lot of cytokines out there, and the research into their effects is new and ongoing. There are several that have shown an association with autoimmune disease, and they have a food link as well; some foods have been shown to increase or decrease certain cytokines. With this in mind, I've tested several foods to test the correlation with arthritis pain.

As mentioned earlier, I've found though testing that the TNFα protein is a leading suspect in autoimmune disease activity. This is backed up by evidence by drug manufacturers, since a main strategy in managing autoimmune disease through medication is by TNFα-antagonistic drugs. Accordingly, the foods that suppress TNFα, like goldenberries, pomegranate, glycine rich foods and garlic, all showed good results in lowering arthritic pain. Fruit like pomegranate runs contrary to a ketogenic diet due to its sugar content, but I consistently felt good eating even large quantities. Goldenberries carry a smaller serving of sugar and seemed even more effective; in fact, when I added them back to my diet, I was able to see a reduction in pain every time.

Goldenberries and garlic both showed efficacy, but there are other features that might be at play, not just inhibiting TNFα. Garlic contains allicin which has been shown to suppress the HLA-B27 gene, making it specifically beneficial for AS. Both foods show an ability to activate the cytokine IL-10. IL-10 is a complicated animal, acting both inflammatory and anti-inflammatory. IL-10 represses other proteins like TNFα, and IL-10 overexpression can lead to immunosuppression, effectively calming an already overactive immune response. Not all studies indicate a benefit, as one study showed that treatment with IL-10 in clinical trials did not significantly benefit patients with RA. However, the Epstein-Barr virus (EBV), the virus that has come up several times in my research and that I tested positive for, has been shown to be structurally similar to IL-10 and the virus may use this similarity to evade the immune system. AS patients have been found to have a hypersensitivity to EBV, and an even greater hypersensitivity in patients with RA. Do we also have a hypersensitivity to IL-10? There is also the tested observation that HIV-positive patients tend to suffer fewer AS symptoms. IL-10 is upregulated during HIV infection, so does it follow that IL-10 reduces inflammation in AS patients?

When in doubt, we must look at test data. IL-10 can be upregulated through calorie restriction, sun exposure, exercise, regular sleep and diet. While it's difficult to say if any of these provided benefit specifically through IL-10 upregulation, I can say that they all made me feel less pain. Since they are all natural solutions we should be using anyway, I can't help but recommend them, even calorie restriction, which has shown to provide numerous other health benefits in autoimmune disease, cancer, diabetes and obesity.

As for IL-17, studies show that sulfasalazine suppresses the HLA-B27 gene through IL-17, and some compounds like ursolic acid, found in apple peel and most fruit peels, and in herbs like rosemary, can inhibit IL-17, providing the same benefit as the medication, albeit to a milder effect. IL-23 is a mediator of inflammation and generally correlated with IL-17. Another study shows that DHA, found in fish oil, and epigallocatechin gallate, found in green tea, could modulate these pro-inflammatory cytokines. A reduction in IL-17 has recently been shown to increase boldness in mice (Yeager, 2020) and an increase is suspect for increased anxiety and depression in humans. This all seems to correlate with the heightened inflammatory condition that comes with high IL-17 and AS symptoms.

**Epstein-Barr virus**

A month after the onset of my ankylosing spondylitis, I was tested for EBV, which is the best-known cause of mononucleosis, also known as "mono" for short or the "kissing disease." I tested positive for the virus, although my GP explained that it's difficult to tell how long ago the infection occurred. During the onset of AS, I had symptoms consistent with mononucleosis, so it may have occurred then and precipitated my AS. However, an investigation concluded that *"patients with AS, like those with RA, show a B cell defect"* and further study showed that patients with AS show a hyper-responsiveness to EBV, not as extreme as patients with RA, but more reactive than a healthy individual. (V.R. Windor, 1987) Another report by R. Dengler indicates that mononucleosis can increase your risk for autoimmune diseases in general. The EBV is a very common virus, 90% of Americans have it, and *"children infected with EBV are up to 50 times more likely to eventually develop lupus"* an autoimmune disease not dissimilar from AS. The physiology behind the connection is unclear, but the correlation is strong. Another study suggests that the autoimmune response is induced by EBV in various types of arthritis and Crohn's disease (J H Vaughan, 1995). In the case of AS, it may be related to the HLA-B27 gene, which predisposes a person to develop AS after contact with EBV, such as biomimicry, or there may be another mechanism. (Cavallini, 2018) My situation is consistent with EBV being a cause or a contributor to the onset of AS.

## Dietary starch and inflammation

Starch is a naturally occurring part of many foods. It's a polysaccharide, or a carbohydrate that plants use to store energy, and it provides us with food energy. It's a large number of sugar molecules bonded together to produce one large molecule, and our bodies break down various types of starch back into sugars that we can use as energy. Some starches are undigestible but are consumed as food by the bacteria in our gut. Other starches pass through our systems untouched.

### *Rapidly digested starch – simple starches and sugars*

Amylopectin is a large starch molecule (actually a polysaccharide), with a structure made up of millions of glucose molecules that branch out and form a crystalline structure. Its glucose units are easily broken apart by enzymes during digestion, which makes it, by definition, a rapidly digestible starch. Because amylopectin is so easy for the body to break down into simple sugars, it can boost your blood sugar and spike your insulin levels. Typically, the vegetarian foods that we eat are 70%-80% amylopectin, with the rest of the starch content coming from amylose starch. An example of a food that has all its starch content made up from amylopectin starch is glutinous rice. When testing this in my diet, I was able to tolerate this type of starch. However, it was noticeably a high-glycemic index food and it gave me rosacea. Even though these foods are not always the healthiest, especially if you are trying to watch your weight or if you have diabetes, they do not always seem to have a direct impact in causing AS, although high-GI foods are generally considered inflammatory and may contribute to autoimmune disease in general. Oligosaccharides like maltodextrin, or simple sugars like monosaccharides, can also be placed in this category as they are easily digested into sugars, or are themselves already simple sugars.

*Indigestible starches*

At the opposite end of the spectrum are indigestible starches, like fibre, that pass through us completely. These include natural cells from plants such as cellulose (a polysaccharide) or inulin and provide health benefit to us by providing bulk to our stool, even though we obtain no nutrients or energy from it. These types of starches are not a concern with AS or autoimmune disease in general. They are most certainly recommended for all disease conditions.

*Resistant starch*

Resistant starch, or slowly digested starch (also a polysaccharide) include starches that cannot be digested by us, since our enzymes, like amylase, cannot split the molecule into smaller sugar molecules. Resistant starch is insoluble but will be consumed and fermented by bacteria in the colon. This fermentation is often the source of flatulence. Dietary sources include green bananas (not black, very ripened bananas because the starch in the banana has already converted to sugar), potatoes, legumes, grains and corn.

In these foods, the starch we primarily need to concern ourselves within the context of AS is called amylose. Amylose contains 500 to 20,000 molecules of glucose connected together in a straight chain. The chain twists into a helix and then two chains bond together, forming a structure that resists the digestive enzymes trying to break the glucose molecules apart. As a result, amylose is slowly digested (by the amylase enzyme) and absorbed, which is why it's called a slowly digestible starch. Amylose would be normally good for you because it is digested slowly and releases sugar to your body slowly, avoiding spikes in insulin or blood sugar. In persons with AS, in my own experience tracking dietary changes and the experience I've heard from others, **amylose in the diet is a primary contributor to arthritis flares and increased pain.**

## Starch and Klebsiella

> *"When AS is involved, the argument to control the disease through diet is even more compelling, based on recent studies that link the Klebsiella Pnumoniae bacteria with the disease." (Taha Rashid, 2013)*

How does starch in our diet contribute to arthritis? *Klebsiella pneumoniae* is a relatively common bacteria that exists in the colons of many people. It can produce pullulanase enzymes that can cleave hard starch molecules that can't be digested by the human digestive system, and it uses these molecules as food to survive the digestive tract. So, amylose starch in the diet allows *Klebsiella* to survive and thrive in the colon. And I mean thrive.

A study by Dr. A. Ebringer showed that 45 subjects, divided into low and high-carbohydrate diet groups, showed significant counts of *Klebsiella* in their feces, with the high-carbohydrate group showing 30,000 per gram, which was 42 times more than the low carbohydrate group, showing 700 per gram. And while starch may be the main culprit in feeding *Klebsiella*, tests has shown that *Klebsiella* will thrive on simple carbohydrates as well, including sucrose, lactose and glucose, so any overeating or fast transit times of food through the digestive system that can deliver undigested carbohydrates to the colon may contribute to their growth.

The colonization of *Klebsiella* in the colon of AS patients has been observed and noted, so we know it's occurring. Now how does it cause a problem for the patient? As mentioned before, AS has a strong genetic component, associated with HLA-B27 gene. It just so happens that the HLA-B27 antigen (the molecule produced in the body based on the instructions from the HLA-B27 gene) looks a lot like *Klebsiella*. This is called biomimicry. It is believed that the body produces antibodies to attack *Klebsiella* when it is introduced in the body, and once this process starts, these antibodies also begin to react with the body's own joint tissues, essentially being attacked by the immune system as well. (P L Schwimmbeck 1, 1988)

*Klebsiella* is a Gram-negative bacterium, and tests on rats have been conducted where endotoxins from Gram-negative bacteria were injected into rats, which induced uveitis similar to what is seen in AS. (James T. Rosenbaum, 2011) There is a list of hypotheses that are still being investigated to determine the link between HLA-B27, *Klebsiella*, and AS, but there is definitely a correlation.

> *Klebsiella acts through the lower intestine, which explains why fasting and diet may stop AS symptoms if the bacteria is destroyed in the intestine. (A1., 1992)*

There are also studies showing that the absence of germs prevents the development of both gut and joint inflammation in rats with

HLA-B27. Not only does this support the theories above, that *Klebsiella* is part of the problem, but it also suggests a pathway through the gut, since gut inflammation is a factor, with Crohn's disease and ulcerative colitis being associated with AS. (M Hvatum†, The gut–joint axis: cross reactive food antibodies in rheumatoid arthritis, 2006)

To take this gut connection further, another study shows that levels of IgM and IgA antibodies in the intestine are higher in AS patients, and levels of those antibodies correspond with levels of disease activity. When AS is active in the body, there's evidence the body is trying to fight some sort of bacterial invasion in the gut. And it's the bacteria in the gut, not the food itself, because the same study showed that the IgM antibodies in AS patients are not any more reactive to dietary antigens. This is also supported by the fact that sulfasalazine is often effective in treating AS, since sulfasalazine has been shown to reduce IgM levels. (M Hvatum†, The gut–joint axis: cross reactive food antibodies in rheumatoid arthritis, 2006)

## Is starch feeding a monster?

A very important link was discovered by Dr. Ebringer that showed that antigens from the gut microbiota, rather than food, are apparently involved in AS (as opposed to rheumatoid arthritis, which seems to have several different mechanisms of action). In fact, there are now a wealth of studies that show various bacteria, such as *Yersinia*, *Salmonella* or *Klebsiella*, can trigger various types of arthritis and disease, including AS, Reiter's disease, reactive arthritis, psoriatic arthritis and others. The second key to this puzzle is that undigested starch in the gut is suspected to act as food for these bacteria, particularly *Klebsiella*, allowing it to proliferate and increase arthritis symptoms.

Reading Dr. Ebringer's research, and several cases of others attesting to the effects of starch, I was fairly convinced that starch is a major contributing cause of AS. However, I started coming across people claiming the NSD (no-starch diet) didn't work for them, so I decided to look at it more closely. I discovered that there was a simple way to test the content of starch in foods by placing a drop of iodine on a sample of food. Working from personal experience, I listed all the foods that I had tested for starch using iodine testing and tested in my diet for an arthritic reaction. Nearly all the foods I had tested were consistent with the starch theory, except for a couple major outliers.

The first was flour. Since flour is made from wheat, I expected this product to contain amylose starch. My wife made her traditional gingerbread cookies for Christmas of 2017 and I really wanted to enjoy some, so I took a risk and tried them out. I tried the cookies (way too many of them, but this was a good thing for the sake of testing) and I didn't have any reaction! This flour turned black when tested with iodine, indicating amylose starch. Now I was really confused, How could the flour contain amylose starch but be tolerated in my diet? Was the starch/*Klebsiella* theory incorrect? Researching further, I found that the particular brand of flour I was using had added amylase. I discovered that amylase is a natural enzyme that is added to the flour to break down the starches into simple sugars for the yeast to consume when making bread. Were the starch molecules being broken down before they could reach my gut as food for *Klebsiella*? Perhaps this was the reason I was able to tolerate it? I retested the flour in my diet, but this time for a longer period. Day one, I added the flour to a homemade bread, and I passed day one with no reaction. On day two, I added a larger quantity of the bread to my diet, and I started to see a reaction. There was redness across my toes, and swelling, especially in one particular toe that had previously showed dactylitis. On day three I added more bread, and this time it was made with yeast (I had previously made the bread with baking powder instead of yeast, which also turned black during iodine testing) and some pizza crust made with yeast and wheat flour. This is when things really flared up. I had pain in both heels, my toes were showing more swelling, and my hands and wrists were now starting to show stiffness. It lasted overnight, but fortunately it started to quiet down the next day. The cause of this inflammation may still be debatable, as white flour is a food with a high glycemic index and will be generally inflammatory for this reason alone, but it does seem to fit the evidence that some residual amounts of amylose starch may have contributed to the inflammation through my gut.

## Amylase supplementation

The concept intrigued me, and I was curious to experiment with amylase further. I was able to find a good quality amylase supplement. I thought if I could test some suspect starchy foods, with and without amylase, I could collect more evidence that starch is the problem and find a solution at the same time.

During my Thanksgiving Day dinner, I went heavy on the foods containing flour in the form of pie crust. Also, I ate some yogurt that contained tapioca starch, which iodine tested black. Day one, I was doing fine. The second day, I had another slice of pie, and then cheese on a slice of whole-grain bread and two bites of banana. I was nervous about the bread. I had had a very clear and severe flare-up in the past when finishing my son's whole wheat toast. Unfortunately, the amylase enzyme did not protect me from the toast. A couple hours later, my back and neck began to get sore, and my neck was sore enough to cause a headache. I developed pain under my chin and my sternum became sore. According to my daily log, this was the worst flare-up in the past 112 days. I didn't do any other activity or eat any other food out of the norm that I could find to explain the flare-up. Fortunately, it subsided quickly; the next morning I was down to a scale 2 out of 10 on the pain scale (from scale 4 out of 10 after the bread) and to about scale 1 in the afternoon, after about 17 hours of fasting.

I was disappointed. I had hoped that amylase enzymes might provide a protective effect against these foods, at least partially. Interestingly, and like in previous tests, I did fine on refined white flour, until I added whole wheat bread. A clear distinction, but why? Amylose starch will pass through the stomach and provide food for *Klebsiella*, while amylopectin starch will digest. Was it a ratio between these starches in flour, or the digestibility of the whole grain? After a week of recovery, I was willing to experiment again the following weekend. Limiting myself to the refined white flour, and doubling the dose of amylase enzyme, I was able to tolerate the starch on an ongoing basis. It seemed as though the amylase enzymes had helped, but I was still limited to the overall quantity of amylose in my diet.

In a way, however, it seemed like the whole investigation into amylase was in vain. It took me so long to find a way to work starch back into my diet that I had gotten used to not eating it, and I realized how much better I feel and function without it. Occasionally, perhaps on the holidays, it's nice to know I can enjoy a slice of pie if I'm cautious with the ingredients, but on a day-to-day basis, I don't desire flour products and I feel just fine without them. Life seems better and easier just avoiding them now that I was used to a more vegetable-based diet, which is a diet recommended for healthy living anyway.

## Inflammation, gut health perspective

I most definitely noticed a connection between my gut health and my arthritis pain. While starch seemed to have a clearly causative role, the level of general stress I put my gut through, seemed to have a contributing role. For example, I could get away with eating some inflammatory foods if starch was clearly avoided. Starch would cause problems, but starch and inflammatory foods combined were worse. I realized there were multiple lines of attack I needed to take to keep AS under control, that included lowering inflammation and allowing joint healing, in addition to avoiding starch to avoid flare-ups. At least one study suggests that the breach of the intestinal barrier by external antigens may lead to a list of immune responses. (Qinghui Mu, 2017) If patients with compromised immune systems can be more susceptible to *Klebsiella* infection, this suggests that once infection is reduced and under control, focus should be placed on minimizing inflammatory foods and strengthening the immune system.

In fact, there is now plenty of evidence that shows inflammation in the gut can exacerbate a number of health issues, including arthritis and cancer, and it has its own host of problems, like Crohn's disease or ulcerative colitis.

## Digestive system health

In my personal experience with AS, the arthritis pain was preceded by cramps and diarrhea, and always showed correlation to gut health. Since these symptoms were experienced at the onset of the disease and before medications were prescribed, it suggested to me that there was an underlying, pre-existing cause related to the digestive system.

I had a second phase of diarrhea, although this was somewhat expected, as I read it is often a side effect of moving to a low-carb diet. The symptom did feel very different then the stomach problems I experienced at the onset of the disease. This time, it was not accompanied with fever, headache, chills or extreme lethargy, but it did include bloating, flatulence, and sometimes major discomfort after dinner. I may have been getting used to eating vegetables at every meal, which is something we should all get used to doing anyway. Over a period of about two weeks, the diarrhea and bloating subsided and I began to feel much better on my new diet. Part of this may have been a result of eating more typical serving sizes, which I believe helped reduce bloating. Before my change in diet, I would always eat large portion sizes and often received jokes about having a hollow leg where I could store all the food I ate, because it didn't really show otherwise. Now, with my arthritis pains mostly subsided, and a stable, mostly vegetable and fish diet, I feel that my digestive system has healed greatly. I don't have the same problems as I did before, and I have no use for antacids. The correlation between arthritis and gut health showed itself again as my diet took effect over the months. The bloating, diarrhea and flatulence all decreased in conjunction with reduced arthritis pain and inflammation, and they were eliminated right around the same time my arthritis pains were completely eliminated. On several occasions, when I did overeat and flatulence and bloating returned, it would often be accompanied by a return in back, neck and foot pain.

## Purging bacteria from the colon – an accidental but telling experiment

During the 2017 Christmas holidays, about one-and-a-half years after the onset of my symptoms, I was off all medication, doing my best to manage my diet, and still dealing with occasional minor flare-ups. I attended a Christmas party with my wife. It was a party thrown by one of my customers, so it was a little bit stressful because I wanted the night to go well. I was experiencing my latest flare-up in my heel and foot that evening, but it was nothing too serious, more of a nuisance. A day later, my wife was feeling nausea and bloating, and she had a headache and diarrhea. A day later, I had some major bloating, gas and diarrhea. Since it hit us both, we suspected some sort of food poisoning. The diarrhea lasted about three days, and my body flushed out everything it had. The usual BRAT diet (bananas, rice, applesauce, and toast) that you might eat to help alleviate diarrhea was mostly of no use to me, since those are starchy foods, so I stuck to apple and kefir, since I read that diarrhea purges both good and bad bacteria, and that it's important to replenish the good. This bout of sickness completely cleared up my arthritis symptoms for over a week, including overnight stiffness that I was still experiencing nightly. This experience seemed to fit the theory of *Klebsiella* in the gut being the cause of the arthritis.

A second experience of this "arthritis benefit from a bowel purge" occurred in February 2018. It was less drastic than the case during the Christmas holidays, but still showed a very clear correlation. On February 25, 2018, I may have eaten something that disagreed with me—I could never determine the exact cause—but next morning I had some early morning diarrhea and a spike in lower-back pain. This back pain had been present for the past few days, but it seemed the most severe on this particular morning. I had another movement later that morning at 9:00 a.m. and with it, my lower-back pain suddenly cleared. It was so immediate that I suspect pressure on the spine may have been a factor, but the pain relief was lasting.

This second occurrence triggered a review my log for any other correlations, and I noticed the same pattern on February 22 (the morning after too many prunes, and the same morning I experienced some general arthritis relief and complete flexibility in my wrists for the first time) and possibly some correlation on February 9, but this occurrence was difficult to be sure about because I had introduced some new foods at the time. Another clear correlation was recorded on August 14 of the same year, when a noticeable and immediate reduction in heel pain occurred. The night before, I had eaten a good amount of peanut butter (something I was trying to phase out at the time due to its omega-6 content, but I just couldn't resist) and a good amount of kefir, which may have gotten my bowel flora moving. Interestingly, there was no pain relief in my second toe, which, in hindsight, showed symptoms of being a strain-related injury and not related to the arthritis.

## Overeating

Overeating has been a big problem for me, though you wouldn't notice just by looking at me. Before my AS diagnosis, I was a big binge eater. When eating with a group, I always received the comments that I must have a hollow leg; somewhere to store all the food I just ate. I could eat a very big meal without it really showing, although I would have to occasionally loosen my belt a couple notches. My body mass index (BMI) was usually 26. At 5'10-3/4" and 180 lbs, I was technically overweight, but I never considered myself as such; I was always athletic, on the muscular side, and so I always assumed that the BMI score was just a result of carrying a little more muscle mass. As a result, I always allowed myself to eat as much as I wanted. I had avoided any red meat since I was a teenager, but I loved my starchy foods: sandwiches, pasta, pizza, packaged cereals, waffles, and cake. Often, I would eat myself into a food coma; a big pasta lunch that would knock me out by 2:00 p.m. Maybe some people do this to themselves during a big, Thanksgiving turkey dinner, but for me it was a regular occurrence. Often on weekends, I would go for a four- to six-hour hike, then have a pizza and cake to treat myself for the hike. A birthday cake. No birthday, just me and cake.

During the onset of my AS, this may have been one of the conditions that set myself up for the onset of the disease. If *Klebsiella* does in fact play its part in the development of the disease, I consumed plenty of amylose starch to allow it to proliferate. My bowel was primed to support *Klebsiella*. Once AS was established, I noticed on several occasions that overeating, being inflammatory on its own, could cause an increase in arthritic pain. I loved the feeling of being "full," so when I had to cut out bread and pasta, I stuffed myself on cabbage and other vegetables, and even stuck to foods that I knew caused no reaction in smaller quantities, but they still caused problems when my stomach felt stretched. Occasionally, I would eat my dinner, then head back to the kitchen to see what I could eat next. Once I was satisfied, I would continue eating. Once I was full, I would snack a little more until I felt bloated. Once I felt bloated, I would see what else I could fit in before bedtime. The nights that I did this, I would suffer for it overnight and the next morning, in multiple ways, such as experiencing bloating, diarrhea, and arthritic pain. I was your typical "feasting" type of eater. So, I shouldn't have been surprised that when I started intermittent fasting, skipping my breakfast was not such a challenge—even a 24-hour fast until the next dinner was not so difficult—but once I started eating, I found it very hard to stop.

Once I developed a bit of discipline around my serving sizes, I found it helped greatly, especially around dinner time. There are a few strategies around eating habits that have worked well for me.

I learned self-control and to practise restraint when it comes to food. I made a conscious effort to make a change. I learned to set my portion size. Setting all my food on a plate and sitting down to a proper meal helped establish a pattern on what a proper portion size should be, instead of eating straight out of the fridge or eating nuts out of a bag. I began to drink water after a meal. Normally, I still felt hungry after a meal, but if I waited half-an-hour, and especially if I drank some water, it would hit my stomach, I would get that full feeling, and I would realize how much I just ate. Out of sight, out of mind; I became especially proficient at putting away leftovers right after a meal, so I would avoid finishing what was left, including my kids' leftovers that were staring me in the face, calling my name . . .

I managed my boredom. When I started fasting, one challenge was that I would get bored! Preparing and eating food takes up a lot of time—it's a social convention we share with friends and family—but only when I started fasting did I realize how often I eat just for something to do. I would eat not because my body needed nourishment, or even because I felt hungry, I would eat just because I enjoyed eating. And sometimes I wouldn't even enjoy it; I would binge eat and barely pay attention to what I was eating while it was going down my throat. Just a bad habit; something to do. This is apparently triggered by our body's need for dopamine; a way to wake us up and create some excitement or something rewarding. Certainly, I've found that keeping busy makes overeating easier to avoid. It's easy to take my mind off food when I'm doing something else, especially when it's something more interesting than the cold leftovers I could be inhaling. Getting out of the kitchen and doing something else for about an hour after eating, until the urge to snack was gone, helped. For me, going into the garage with the radio on or finishing some other chores worked well. Another example is taking a walk or doing some light or moderate physical activity after a meal. It aids with digestion and reducing that stuffed feeling.

I identified the psychological stresses in my life and found healthy ways of coping, and not with food. On the IF diet, I feared not having enough calorie intake, or experiencing fatigue the next day, so I would intentionally overeat. I spread meals out during the course of the day. I learned not to try to skip one meal and decide to cover up on the next. This can be a balancing act if I'm intermittent fasting as well, since it's also beneficial to go for a good portion of the day without eating. For me, an eating window between 4:00 p.m. and 8:00 p.m. worked well.

I avoided large servings of grains. Since I was avoiding starch already, there were only a few grains or flours that I could eat, but I initially missed breads so much that I nearly made up for it with other grains, like almond flour, coconut flour, flax, chia, or lower-starch substitutes like amaranth flour. They were all healthy foods, but I started to notice that eating grains wouldn't make me feel full until about an hour later. By then, I would have eaten a lot, and even though I decided to stop eating, I continued to feel fuller. And thirsty. And of course, drinking water made me feel fuller. By then it was far too late, and on many occasions I was so bloated that I felt like throwing up.

How does this all relate? As mentioned before, *Klebsiella*, a suspected cause of AS and source of inflammation in other autoimmune diseases, feeds from the amylose starch in our diet. But overeating can increase digestive transit times, and introduce undigested simple carbohydrates, which can provide food for *Klebsiella*, with the result being just as bad as consuming starch.

# CHAPTER 5

# KLEBSIELLA

### Treatment by controlling Klebsiella

> *Low starch, low carbs, and moderate sized meals will help reduce Klebsiella bacteria in gut, will reduce Klebsiella antibodies produced by the body, which will help reduce the act of biomimicry with the HLA-B27 gene. (Taha Rashid, 2013)*

Cellulose from plant fibres, inulin or other indigestible fibre is not an issue because studies of *Klebsiella* have shown that it will not grow on this type of substrate, nor on protein or fats, and instead will grow on simple sugars. Sugars can appear in the gut through fast transit times, undigested food, or by the breakdown of amylose starch in the gut by *Klebsiella*. The key to this strategy is limiting the food available to *Klebsiella* to keep its growth under control. One other study showed that there was a significant increase in intestinal bacteria in general with diets (in rats) containing resistant potato starch when compared to those taking rapidly digestible waxy maize starch. (Taha Rashid, 2013)

Amylopectin starch (which is easily digestible) did not cause me any arthritis flare-ups. I experimented with glutinous rice, which contains amylopectin but not amylose. I was able to tolerate this in my diet with no correlation to arthritis pain or flare-up, although I did experience rosacea on several occasions, as if I were eating a bowl of sugar. I typically felt best when I kept the quantity of glutinous rice low, and I generally felt better eliminating it from my diet altogether.

## Calculating starch

There is also a way to calculate the amount of starch in your food—from the nutrition label—but be warned that this is total starch, which could be amylose or amylopectin. Total carbohydrates listed on the nutrition label (in Canada) is the sum of dietary fibre, plus sugars (yes, sugars are carbs) with the remainder of the total coming from starches. For example, a label with 37 g of total carbs, with 4 g of fibre and 1 g of sugar, means the food will have 32 g of starch (37 - 4 - 1 = 32). What type of starch? Refer to the ingredients list and research your foods. For example, most of the starch in chia will be resistant starch, which can feed the healthy bacteria in your gut and act as a prebiotic. The opposite end of the spectrum can be something like white rice, which contains a lot of rapidly digestible starch, which your body easily breaks down into sugars.

## Iodine testing your food for starch – Don't feed Klebsiella!

Very conveniently, there is an easy and inexpensive test you can do at home to test your foods for the starch that is believed to be a concern for AS. It's a simple test, however, there are some points to be made to ensure an accurate result.

Potassium iodide, which can often be purchased for under $10 at your local pharmacy, can be dropped onto a small quantity of food for testing. The food will only turn blue/black in the presence of amylose, not amylopectin. If amylase starch is not present, the mixture will stay brown.

This test is more specific than a check for starch content, since it tests specifically for amylose starch content. Due to the linkages in the amylose molecule, amylose produces a spiral shape, which is just the right shape for an iodine molecule to fit inside. When this occurs, the iodine reacts with the amylose and the iodine solution turns from yellow/brown to purple/black. It's a clear, visual indicator that amylose is present. This does not occur with amylopectin since the molecule is not soluble in water, and it is not physically the right shape to react with the iodine in this same fashion. This is also true for cellulose or disaccharides like sucrose or fructose. It is a true test to detect only amylose.

First, potassium iodide is very sensitive to the presence of amylose, and it will turn colour even with low fractions of amylose. (Charles, 2003) The test will not show how much amylose is present in the food, which is important because higher quantities of amylose clearly have a greater impact on arthritis. This may depend on your personal situation, but I have been able to tolerate moderate quantities of low-amylose foods.

Secondly, the potassium iodide and starch need to combine, and this can be difficult with solid or dry foods. In my initial testing, I found some foods don't change colour or change colour only after some time (15 minutes). When I added a little bit of water to the solution to help the amylose dissolve, it would turn to black immediately. Because of this lack of mixing, I incorrectly identified some foods as starch free during initial testing. For example, I tested some packaged (dry), oat-based cereal with a drop of iodine. I typically crush the food on a small plate to allow the iodine to mix in. As it contained oats, I was sure it should be turning black, but it stayed brown, and only after a few minutes, only the edges of some of the food pieces turned black. After adding a drop of water and making a small solution, the entire solution immediately turned black, indicating the presence of the amylose starch, which was consistent with my testing of other oat products. This cereal also caused me an overnight flare-up in my foot, which is why I had been testing it and was initially surprised to see it stayed brown.

A third important point is the impact of vitamin C in the mixture. Iodide (in the form of potassium iodide, the form that can be commonly purchased) will react with hydrogen peroxide (also known as a free radical) to produce iodine. Vitamin C, acting as an antioxidant, will convert iodine back to iodide when it has reacted with vitamin C; it is "tied up" and no longer reacts with the amylose starch. If the vitamin C is used up in the solution, the remaining iodide will react with amylose and turn purple. This reaction could also contribute to a delay in colour change, so be sure to take this into consideration when testing foods.

I was initially skeptical of this test, but it proved true time and again as I developed my diet. Often, I didn't understand the link until I tested all the food in my diet. For example, I tested chia and it tested brown, but I felt better when I cut it out of my diet, only to discover later that the cashew milk I used to soak the chia, which I previously assumed was safe, turned black and ended up being the culprit. Chia when soaked in kefir or water caused no reaction.

I highly recommend using this test for foods you eat, especially any packaged or store-bought foods. Often, starches are added to the most surprising places like sour cream, cream cheese, deserts, sauces, sausages and multi-vitamins.

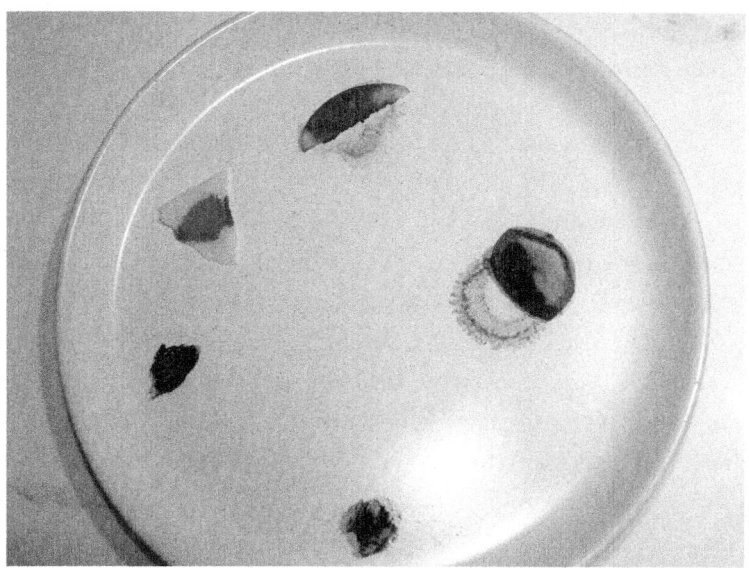

*Testing foods with potassium iodide. Shown from the twelve o'clock position in a clockwise direction: apple turning slightly black over time, banana turning sharply black, oats turning black, sourdough bread turning black, and Swiss cheese staying brown.*

## Foods to avoid that feed Klebsiella

Through my testing, I've compiled a list of foods containing amylose starch that should be avoided if one is trying to avoid feeding *Klebsiella*. By no means is this an exhaustive list, so I recommend you also do your own iodine testing.

In general, all other complex carbs are best limited, since, if combined with a large meal, they may introduce simple sugars to the intestine if undigested material were to pass through. Amylose starch is generally found in legumes, most root vegetables like potatoes, corn, breads and starchy fruits such as bananas. Dietary sugars from moderate amounts of fruit should be plenty, allowing for some fibre and nutrition as well (fructose, glucose, and apparently sucrose have all diet tested ok for me personally, but they may be introduced into the intestine through rapid transit times through the gut caused by overeating).

Fibres that are not a concern include lignin, cellulose, some hemicellulose, chitin (only weakly) and in general, foods that are low in resistant starch, like a high-GI grain such as sticky white rice. This isn't the healthiest advice, but this is what I've observed; I can tolerate a white baguette but a couple slices of "healthy" whole-grain toast have caused severe flare-ups. I've chosen to stay away from bread altogether. Whole grains or seeds that do not iodide test black are ok as a source of non-fermentable, insoluble fibre (they contain lignin, cellulose, some hemicellulose, and chitin), which through my experience, have not caused AS flare-ups. Examples of these foods are chia and flax.

## Resistant starch in foods

With this knowledge at hand, I began testing an assortment of foods, and comparing them to known quantities of amylose, and my reaction to each of the foods. Obtaining quantities of amylose was difficult, as most foods have only their total quantities of starch listed, which may include any combination of amylose and amylopectin. So this also had to be taken into account, as not all high starch foods are high in amylose starch specifically.

The following is a list of foods that I've tested in my diet, tested with iodine, and compared to the reported values of starch content. I've compared these foods to calculated values (again this is total starch, not specifically amylose which appears to be the only one that causes the problem) and listed my results of iodine testing and diet testing (whether or not it caused me a flare).

| Group | Food | Total Starch, Calculated, g/100g | Iodine testing result | Diet testing result | Consistent with starch Theory? |
|---|---|---|---|---|---|
| Beans and lentils | Black beans (canned) | 11.2 | Black | Yes | yes |
| Breads | Naan bread | | Black | Ok in small amounts | Yes |
| Breads | Sourdough | 51.0 | Black | Ok in small amounts | Yes |
| Breads | White rolls | 51.0 | black | Ok in small amounts | Yes |
| Carbonated drinks | Lemonade | 0 | brown | ok | Yes |
| Carbonated drinks | Tonic water | 0 | brown | ok | Yes |
| Cereal, Breakfast | Bran Flakes | 27.6 | Black | not ok | yes |
| Cereal, Breakfast | Corn Bran Squares | 46.7 | | not ok | Yes |
| Cereal, Breakfast | Puffed Rice | 78.6 | Black | not ok | Yes |
| Cheeses | Brie | 0 | brown | ok | yes |
| Cheeses | Cream cheese | 0 | brown | ok | yes |
| Cheeses | Hard cheese (average) | 0 | brown | ok | yes |
| Cheeses | Mozzarella (fresh) | 0 | brown | ok | yes |
| Cheeses | Stilton (blue) | 0 | brown | ok | yes |
| Chicken | Chicken, baked | 0 | brown | ok | yes |
| Duck | Duck, baked | 0 | brown | ok | yes |
| Eggs and egg dishes | Chicken egg, boiled | 0 | brown | ok | Yes |

| Fats and oils | Omega 3 | 0 | Brown | ok | yes |
|---|---|---|---|---|---|
| Fats and oils | Butter | 0 | Brown | ok | Yes |
| Flours, grains and starches | Amaranth flour | 16.9 | Black, delayed with water | ok in small amounts so far | yes |
| Flours, grains and starches | Tapioca (raw) | 95 | Black | Not ok | Yes |
| Flours, grains and starches | Wheat flour | 70.0 | Black, immediate with water | ok in small amounts | yes, explained by Amylase |
| Fresh creams | Heavy cream | 0 | Brown | ok | Yes |
| Fruit, general | Watermelon | 1.3 | Brown | ok | Yes |
| Fruit, general | Apples (raw) | 1.6 | brown | ok | Yes |
| Fruit, general | Avocado (raw) | 1.3 | Brown | ok | yes |
| Fruit, general | Banana, very ripe, completely black skin | 5 | Brown | Ok in small amounts | Yes |
| Fruit, general | Banana, yellow ripe bananas. | 8.4 | Black | not ok | Yes |
| Fruit, general | Blackberries (raw) | 0 | Brown | ok | Yes |
| Fruit, general | Blackcurrents (raw) | 0 | Brown | ok | Yes |
| Fruit, general | Mangoes (ripe, raw) | 0 | Brown | ok | Yes |
| Fruit, general | Clementines | 0 | Brown | ok | Yes |
| Fruit, general | Currants | 0 | Brown | ok | Yes |
| Fruit, general | Dates (raw) | 0 | Brown | ok | Yes |
| Fruit, general | Lemon peel | 0 | Brown | ok | Yes |
| Fruit, general | Prunes (canned in juice) | 0 | Brown | ok | Yes |
| Fruit, general | Goji Berry | 0 | Brown | ok | Yes |

| Fruit, general | Grapes, green | 0.1 | Brown | ok | Yes |
|---|---|---|---|---|---|
| Fruit, general | Kiwi fruit | 0.3 | Brown | ok | Yes |
| Fruit, general | Canteloupe | 0 | Brown | ok | Yes |
| Fruit, general | Nectarines | 0 | Brown | ok | Yes |
| Fruit, general | Olives (in brine) | 0 | Brown | ok | Yes |
| Fruit, general | Oranges | 0.6 | TBD | ok | Yes |
| Fruit, general | Pears (raw) | 0 | Brown | ok | Yes |
| Fruit, general | Pineapple (raw) | 0 | Brown | ok | Yes |
| Fruit, general | Raisins | 16.3 | Brown | ok | Yes |
| Fruit, general | Strawberries (raw) | 0 | brown | ok | Yes |
| Herbs and spices | Parsley (fresh) | 0 | Brown | ok | Yes |
| Juices | Apple juice | 0 | brown | ok | Yes |
| Juices | Pineapple juice | 0 | Brown | ok | Yes |
| Juices | Orange juice | 0 | TBD | ok | Yes |
| Meat and meat products | Chicken, smoked, deli | 15est. | Black | not ok | yes |
| Meat and meat products | Escargo | 2 | black, delayed | ok | Yes |
| Meat and meat products | Ham, Black forest, deli | 1.5 | | ok | yes |
| Meat and meat products | Turkey, smoked, deli | 15est. | Black | not ok | yes |
| Milk and Milk Products | Evaporated milk (whole) | 0 | Brown | ok | Yes |
| Milk and Milk Products | Goats milk (pasteurised) | 0 | TBD | ok | Yes |
| Miscellaneous foods | Chocolate, with soy lethicin | 15est. | black | ok in small amounts | yes |
| Miscellaneous foods | Gelatine | 0 | TBD | ok | Yes |

| | | | | | |
|---|---|---|---|---|---|
| Miscellaneous foods | Mustard, raw organic, smooth | 0 | brown | ok | Yes |
| Miscellaneous foods | Vinegar | 0 | TBD | ok | Yes |
| Nuts and seeds | Almond flour | | Brown | ok | yes |
| Nuts and seeds | Almonds (with skin) | 6.1 | brown | ok | Yes |
| Nuts and seeds | Almonds, blanched | 2.7 | brown | ok | Yes |
| Nuts and seeds | Cashew cream | 12 | Black | not ok | Yes |
| Nuts and seeds | Cashew milk | 20 | Black | not ok | Yes |
| Nuts and seeds | Cashew nuts (roasted and salted) | 20.7 | black, delayed | not ok | Yes |
| Nuts and seeds | Chia seed | 8.0 | Brown | ok | yes |
| Nuts and seeds | Coconut (creamed block) | 0 | TBD | ok | Yes |
| Nuts and seeds | Coconut flour | 0 | Brown | ok | Yes |
| Nuts and seeds | Coconut meat (raw) | 0 | Brown | ok | Yes |
| Nuts and seeds | Coconut milk | 0 | Brown | ok | Yes |
| Nuts and seeds | Flaxseed | 0.4 | brown | ok | Yes |
| Nuts and seeds | Hazelnuts | 2.7 | brown | ok | Yes |
| Nuts and seeds | Hemp Hearts | 0 | brown | ok | Yes |
| Nuts and seeds | Macadamia nuts (salted) | 0.4 | brown | ok | Yes |
| Nuts and seeds | Nut butter, Cashew, almond | 15est | Black | not ok | No |

| Category | Item | | Colour | | |
|---|---|---|---|---|---|
| Nuts and seeds | Nut Butter, peanut | 6.4 | brown | ok in small amounts | Yes |
| Nuts and seeds | Peanuts (plain) | 10.0 | Black | not ok | Yes |
| Nuts and seeds | Pecan nuts | 0 | Brown | ok | Yes |
| Nuts and seeds | Pilinut | 3est | brown | ok | Yes |
| Nuts and seeds | Pistachio nuts (roasted and salted) | 10.0 | | ok in small amounts | yes |
| Nuts and seeds | Walnuts | 4.4 | Brown | ok | Yes |
| Oils | Coconut oil | 0 | Brown | ok | Yes |
| Oils | Avocado Oil | 0 | brown | ok | yes |
| Oils | Cod liver oil | 0 | Brown | ok | Yes |
| Oils | Ghee (butter) | 0 | TBD | ok | Yes |
| Oils | Olive oil | 0 | TBD | ok | Yes |
| Powdered drinks and essences | Cocoa powder | 23.2 | Brown | ok | Yes |
| Powdered drinks and essences | Coffee | 0 | No | ok | Yes |
| Rice | Sticky Rice (amylopectin) | 19.9 | Black | ok in small amounts | Yes, but why black? |
| Savoury snacks | Popcorn | 7 est. | | ok | yes |
| Seafood | Anchovies (canned in oil, drained) | 0 | brown | ok | Yes |
| Seafood | Cod | 0 | Brown | ok | Yes |
| Seafood | Crab | 0 | Brown | ok | Yes |
| Seafood | Haddock | 0 | TBD | ok | Yes |
| Seafood | Halibut (grilled) | 0 | TBD | ok | Yes |
| Seafood | Herring | 0 | TBD | ok | Yes |
| Seafood | Lemon sole | 0 | TBD | ok | Yes |
| Seafood | Mackerel | 0 | TBD | ok | Yes |
| Seafood | Salmon Jerky | 15 est. | Black | not ok | yes |

| Category | Food | Value | Color | Status | Yes/No |
|---|---|---|---|---|---|
| Seafood | White fish | 0 | Brown | ok | Yes |
| Soups, sauces and miscellaneous foods | Chicken broth | 0 | brown | ok | Yes |
| Soups, sauces and miscellaneous foods | Tomato soup with grated carrot, chicken base | 12 est. | black | not ok | Yes |
| Sugars, syrups and preserves | Honey | 0 | brown | ok | Yes |
| Sugars, syrups and preserves | Icing Sugar | 6.0 | brown | ok but only tested in small amounts | Yes |
| Sugars, syrups and preserves | Syrup (golden) | 0 | brown | ok | Yes |
| Turkey | Roasted (dark meat) | 0 | | ok | Yes |
| Vegetable dishes | Sauerkraut | 0.1 | | ok | Yes |
| Vegetable dishes | Tomato sauce | 0.1 | Brown | ok | Yes |
| Vegetables, general | Artichokes, Globe (boiled) | 0 | brown | ok | Yes |
| Vegetables, general | Asparagus (raw) | 0 | TBD | ok | Yes |
| Vegetables, general | Broccoli (green, raw) | 2.7 | brown | ok | Yes |
| Vegetables, general | Brussel sprouts (raw) | 3 | black | ok | Yes, small quantities |
| Vegetables, general | Cabbage (raw, average) | 0.3 | brown | ok | Yes |

| | | | | | | |
|---|---|---|---|---|---|---|
| Vegetables, general | Carrots | 2.5 | Black | not ok | Yes |
| Vegetables, general | Cauliflower (raw) | 0.4 | brown | ok | Yes |
| Vegetables, general | Celery (raw) | 0 | Brown | ok | Yes |
| Vegetables, general | Cucumber (raw) | 0 | Brown | ok | Yes |
| Vegetables, general | Curly kale (raw) | 0 | Brown | ok | Yes |
| Vegetables, general | Garlic (raw) | 14.7 | TBD | OK in small amounts | Yes |
| Vegetables, general | Mushrooms (white) | 0.2 | brown | ok | Yes |
| Vegetables, general | Onions (raw) | 0 | brown | ok | Yes |
| Vegetables, general | Peppers (capsicum, chilli, green, raw) | 0 | brown | ok | Yes |
| Vegetables, general | Pickled cucumbers (in saltwater) | 0 | brown | ok | Yes |
| Vegetables, general | Pumpkin (raw) | 3.7 | black | ok | yes |
| Vegetables, general | Radish (red, raw) | 0.1 | Brown | ok | yes |
| Vegetables, general | Spaghetti squash | 2.7 | TBD | ok | Yes |
| Vegetables, general | Spouts, onion | 0.1 | brown | ok | Yes |
| Vegetables, general | Spring onions (bulbs and tops, raw) | 0.1 | black | ok | Yes, small quantities |

| Vegetables, general | Tomatoes (raw) | 0.1 | TBD | ok | Yes |
|---|---|---|---|---|---|
| Vegetables, general | Zucchini (raw) | 0 | Brown | ok | Yes |
| Vegetables, general | Iceberg lettuce, raw | 0 | Brown | ok | Yes |
| Vegetables, general | Artichoke | 0 | Brown | ok | Yes |

## Klebsiella bactericidals

A bactericide is a substance that kills bacteria. Some studies have looked at the sensitivity of *Klebsiella* to different foods, to determine if there are any bactericides that will kill *Klebsiella*, and there are a few that show promise. The first, and most effective, is oregano oil. Two phenols that constitute about 78–85% of oregano essential oils (EOs), carvacrol and thymol, have been shown to provide antimicrobial activity against *Klebsiella*. (al. M. F., 2015)

*Klebsiella pneumoniae*, when tested in vitro (in a dish in the lab), showed sensitivity to both thyme (9.5 µg/mL) and oregano EOs (73.5 µg/mL). Most efficient were the EOs from thyme followed by those of oregano. (Maria Fournomiti, 2015)

Side effects are uncommon with thyme teas and tinctures. Very large dosages, such as three or four cups of thyme tea consumed all at once, may occasionally promote nausea and a sensation of warmth and perspiration. The concentrated essential oil, however, is extremely strong and irritating. Pure essential oil of thyme can cause headaches and confusion, due to the presence of the chemical compound thujone. When you use thyme volatile oil, you must dilute it before ingesting it or placing it on the skin to avoid burns and inflammation. Oregano oil is also very potent, and only requires a few drops from a tincture. It produces a burning sensation in the throat and mouth, and I found the easiest way to swallow it was to combine it with a small amount of another oil like olive oil.

Honey is another substance that has been determined to be bactericidal against *Klebsiella*, in vitro. (Merckoll P1, 2009), (Kasa, 2016). Ginger has also been identified as being bactericidal against *Klebsiella*, in vitro. (Tathagat. E. Waghmare*, 2014) However, I personally recommend caution adding ginger to your diet—both ginger root and ginger root boiled to make tea—as both have iodide tested black, indicating they contain amylose starch.

It should be noted that these tests were conducted in vitro and not in vivo (in a real-world, human body setting). So, it is not clear if oregano, thyme or honey carry their effects through the digestive system in sufficient concentration to have an effect on *Klebsiella* in the intestine. I haven't been able to find any studies showing the efficacy of oregano, thyme, honey or ginger against *Klebsiella* in vivo, and I haven't been able to filter out any clear benefits from any of these substances in my diet. Out of the bactericides, my most disciplined testing was with oregano oil, which I took daily for a couple months. I had several other changes in my diet at the time that may have interfered with this test, including cutting out cashews which contain amylose starch. In theory, the oregano oil should have protected me from *Klebsiella* growth despite consuming starch, but it did not seem to have this effect. I experienced several flare-ups while I was regularly consuming oregano oil.

# CHAPTER 6

# FASTING TO REDUCE INFLAMMATION

I was never one to fast, and it was never something I enjoyed. Looking back at my habits before the onset of my arthritis, I always kept myself in a fed state. I would have a large breakfast (usually processed cereal with banana, a healthy but starchy fruit) early in the morning, snacks mid-morning, a big lunch that usually left me tired in the afternoon, an afternoon snack, dinner with the family—I would finish my kids' plates—then of course they would want a bowl of cereal before bed, so I would eat one with them and finish their bowls so I wouldn't have to throw anything out. If not that, I would make waffles loaded with peanut butter and jam before bed. Not only was I never hungry, but carbs were a staple of every meal in the form of cereal, bread, pasta or pizza. This was normal eating for me, and I never considered the idea of voluntarily allowing myself to go hungry, or fasting for any period of time, until I stumbled upon the fact that our bodies produce some of their own medicines and inflammatory effects while in the fasted state.

## Cortisol

I first received local cortisone injections for my arthritis before I had researched cortisol. Cortisol prevents inflammation in the body by preventing the release of certain substances. It can be applied topically, but in my case and in the case of AS, it is almost always injected directly into the joint, at the site of inflammation. I then learned that cortisol is not always a foreign substance; the body produces its own.

The early fasting stage results in cortisol production which reduces inflammation. It's also a stress hormone, so it's important that the body isn't receiving it all the time, just intermittently. I remember reading about the idea of intermittent fasting a decade ago or so, although then it was simply referred to as the body's natural 24-hour cycle (Garner, 2006, p. P.31). In the early fasting state, cortisol stimulates gluconeogenesis (the formation of glucose), and activates anti-stress and anti-inflammatory pathways. (Peart, 2015) So, I thought, why not try fasting and let my body produce its own cortisol naturally? Gluconeogenesis starts well before the exhaustion of glycogen, so the benefits of cortisol production should occur even before ketone body production. During this research period, I also began to learn about the anti-inflammatory properties of ketone bodies.

## Ketone bodies

Ketone bodies are chemicals, including BHB and hydroxybutyrate, that are produced by the liver when the body's glucose stores begin to run low. It is the body's way of manufacturing glucose from fat. It's completely natural and it doesn't mean that you're starving yourself; it's the body's way of tapping into its stored energy in the form of fat. These ketone bodies have a broad range of wonderful side effects that occur through signalling mechanisms that instruct the body to "rest and digest" and conduct all sorts of repair. And it's not just fasting—this occurs whenever you deplete your body's readily available glucose, which can occur with carbohydrate restrictive diets (a keto diet) or prolonged intense exercise. For example, macrophages (white blood cells involved in inflammation) have their NLRP3 gene turned off by exposure to ketone bodies. (Yun-Hee Youm, 2015)

Why is this beneficial to arthritis patients? The NLRP3 gene is involved in general inflammation, and NLRP3, as well as TFRSF1A (rs4149570) are associated with AS susceptibility. *"In their study, published in the Feb. 16 online issue of Nature Medicine, the researchers described how the compound β-hydroxybutyrate (BHB) directly inhibits NLRP3, which is part of a complex set of proteins called the inflammasome. The inflammasome drives the inflammatory response in several disorders including autoimmune diseases, type 2 diabetes, Alzheimer's disease, atherosclerosis, and autoinflammatory disorders."* (Zhao S1, 2017)

The study team introduced BHB to mouse models of inflammatory diseases caused by NLP3. They found that this reduced inflammation, and that inflammation was also reduced when the mice were given a ketogenic diet, which elevates the levels of BHB in the bloodstream.

> *"Our results suggest that the endogenous metabolites like BHB that are produced during low-carb dieting, fasting, or high-intensity exercise can lower the NLRP3 inflammasome," said Dixit."* (Peart, 2015)

As mentioned earlier, a ketonic diet is a diet very low in sugars and carbohydrates, which depletes the body of readily available glucose, forcing the liver to produce ketone bodies. Like we mentioned before in chapter 4, there is evidence that free radical damage contributes to inflammatory joint damage. While antioxidants can be used in the diet to scavenge free radicals, ketone bodies can also work in our favour in this area.

Studies have shown that ketone bodies in a low-carb diet may offer therapeutic potential in a variety of different common and rare disease states, including diseases resulting from free radical damage. (Manninen, 2004), (RL1., 2004) And yes, as discussed earlier, AS, osteoarthritis, and other forms of arthritis are recognized as diseases caused by free radical damage.

Through ketone bodies, apoptosis, and a whole host of other mechanisms, fasting is incredibly protective, reparative, and beneficial for the human body. Studies have even shown that "fasting exerts extensive antitumor effects in various cancers, including colorectal cancer." (al. M.-l. e., 2020) Now that I'm used to fasting, I look forward to it, after a weekend of perhaps too much eating, as a break for my gut to repair and recover, and to reduce my arthritis symptoms along with it.

## Intermittent fasting: Incorporating fasting into your life

It's natural to go for a period of time without eating between dinner and breakfast. Extend this time slightly, say for a period of 16 hours, and it's called intermittent fasting. Starting with a relatively short fast, I shifted my breakfast from 5:30 a.m. to 10:00 a.m. I was going 10:00 p.m. to 10:00 a.m. without food. At the time, 12 hours felt like a long time, but I started to feel the benefits right away. Doing this shortened my morning pain and stiffness period. Eventually, I settled into a 16-hour routine (no eating between 8:00 p.m. and noon the next day). Personally, I felt the most benefit after about 14–16 hours, which is why I settled on this routine. I remember explaining to my family that after 14 hrs, I felt as much benefit as taking a naproxen. The studies seem to support this, since after about 16 hours, especially when combined with a low-carb diet, the body goes into a state of gluconeogenesis (producing its own glucose from protein and fat), which is often associated with ketosis. The body produces more cortisol and ketone bodies which reduce inflammation.

For a person who doesn't like fasting, I also found this to be an easy, regular habit to incorporate into my daily life, without feeling like I was starving myself. I started my intermittent fasting in June of 2017. It's the biggest, single, natural benefit I've felt and it has allowed me to discontinue daily naproxen use. At the time of writing this, I've been continuing with it for about 18 months. I've also extended it to an approximately 19-hour daily fast.

> *"During fasting your body shows a slight shift in the balance of the autonomous nervous system toward the sympathetic side. This so called noradrenergic or adrenergic reaction leads to cold extremities due to less blood flow in the extremities. It also causes the nice feeling of being wide awake and alert. You can enhance (or worsen) the effect by the intake of caffeine (as in coffee). (I have a noticeable feeling of both coldness and alertness after about 14hrs of fasting). The adrenergic response increases corticosterone. Part of the flight/fight response, corticosterone is also linked to anxiety relief and can either facilitate or interrupt conditioned fear." (Dona L. Wong, 2009)*

> *Eating more frequently, reducing evening energy intake, and fasting for longer nightly intervals may lower systemic inflammation (Catherine R. Marinac, 2015).*

> *Fasting is known to decrease intestinal permeability, thus making the gut "less leaky." This may be one of the reasons fasting has been shown to dramatically benefit patients with rheumatoid arthritis (Scand J Rheumatol 1982;11(1):33-38).*

More recently, I've been adding a 5:2 diet cycle of fasting to my routine, which incorporates two, non-consecutive fasting days a week of 600 calories per day for men, and 500 calories per day for women. This diet became popular through the book, *The Fast Diet*, and the BBC documentary by the same name, written by Michael Mosley and Mimi Spencer. I cannot recommend this book enough; it reviews some of the clear benefits for fasting including weight loss, reducing inflammation, improving insulin sensitivity and many other health benefits.

Before long, intermittent fasting along with the occasional longer fast has put me right in the centre of my normal BMI index, a solid 20–24 lbs lighter than I was two years ago. Experimenting with a fasting schedule that suits your life is critical. It needs to be a lifestyle change that you will do on a daily basis, because if you don't do it then you won't receive any benefit. I'm still experimenting with works best for me, but I've already fallen into a comfortable routine with 16:8 daily fasting which has transitioned to 20:4 fast on weekdays, and I'm actually enjoying the weekly or twice-weekly 24-hour fast. The occasional hunger pangs pass relatively easily with some practise, and I feel good near the end of the fast, and even better the next full feeding day. For a while, I tended to overeat a little, but nowhere close enough to compensate for my fast day, and my body feels stronger, like a recovery after a workout. After having a long conversation about fasting with my GP, she recommends both these time frames and considers them both generally safe.

While I'm still experimenting with the amount of fasting that works best for me, I can confidently say that fasting has produced a clear reduction on inflammation as it relates to arthritis.

## Fasting for longer durations

I'd like to start by defining what I would define as long-duration fasting. Longer-term fasting should be defined as anything too long that can't be done sustainably, regularly, or in other words, intermittently. One could do regular, daily, intermittent fasting for as long as about 23 hours a day. This has been called "one meal a day" (OMAD) fasting. In practice, I find the maximum, comfortable, daily intermittent fasting is 22:2 (22 hours fasting by about a 2-hour feeding window), which gives me enough time to eat enough calories without rushing my eating and making myself feel bloated or uncomfortable. So, long-duration fasting could be defined as 24 hours or longer.

There are a few different lengths of water fasts that I've used. All the fasts I did were while I was also doing 16:8 IF, which means if I would skip a day of eating, my last meal would be dinner on, say, a Monday, not eat on Tuesday, and resume my intermittent fasting on Wednesday at noon, giving me a 40-hour fast.

### *Feedback from my doctors*

I tried to be cautious. I didn't want to do myself harm. The general reaction I received from friends when I mentioned fasting was something like, "Three days without food, but won't you die?" I wanted to check with my doctors for some professional opinions. My general practitioner had no problem with a 24-hour, or even 48-hour fast. She recommended some bone broth, but generally suggested to keeping it to this length as it would be very low risk. I suspected maybe since she was Hindu, she might have more cultural exposure to fasting and was more comfortable with the concept of fasting then most in Western culture. I asked my cardiologist. At the time, he was investigating my very slow heartbeat (which I suspect was just from cycling every day) and a second degree atrioventricular (AV) block of the heart. Despite this, he said fasting would be no problem. Fasts longer than this generally are recommended to be medically supervised.

### Forty-hour fast

Forty-hour fasts are great experiences. Usually, once I would reach about 34 hours into the fast, typically at 6:00 a.m., when I would normally wake up to my typical morning stiffness and pain, I would instead feel 100%. Nearly every time in my daily log, I would write to myself "Fasting, the miracle cure!" Except that it wasn't.

Invariably, my symptoms would return after the fast was complete, sometimes on my very first refeeding day, which was very frustrating. In retrospect, after some of my earlier fasts, I did a horrible job of refeeding, typically eating the wrong foods and too much, too fast. Despite the healing and pain relief that fasting brought, it was still a temporary solution; I couldn't just stop eating indefinitely.

### Extended fasts, three to seven days

The fasts that are longer than 40 hours, I try to do seasonally, like a reset to the system and an extended healing period. The best way I can describe it is the "rest and digest" period, which is the informal phrase commonly used to describe the body's parasympathetic nervous system, which is responsible for activities in the body such as rest, digestion, increased intestinal and gland activity, and is associated with a lower heart rate. I always experienced the same level of pain relief on the longer fasts, which continued as long as I was fasting, and a good level of energy. I always maintained my typical daily activities, including cycling. It was on the third extended fast that I finally got the refeeding portion right. I always had the tendency to eat way too much, too soon.

During fasting, usually about three to four days in, constipation can set in and at times I've found it severe. A natural fibre, like inulin, has been effective for me without causing any type of starch-related flare.

Page quotes Casey A. Wood, M.D., professor of chemistry in the Medical Department of Bishop's College, Montreal, in an article in the *Canada Medical Record*, entitled "Starvation in the treatment of Acute Articular Rheumatism," as giving the *"history of seven cases where the patients were speedily restored to health by simply abstaining from food from four to eight days, and he says he could have given the history of 40 more from his own practice."* No drugs were used and *"in no case did this treatment fail."* The cases reported *"included men and women of different ages, temperaments, occupations, and social positions."* Dr. Wood says: *"From the quick and almost invariably good results to be obtained by simple abstinence from food, I am inclined to the idea that rheumatism is, after all, only a phase of indigestion."* Dr. Page adds: *"In chronic rheumatism he obtained less positive results, but did not venture to try fasts of longer duration."* Dr. Wood concludes by saying that *"this treatment, obviating as it does, almost entirely, danger of cardiac complications, will be bound to realize all that has been claimed for it — a simple, reliable remedy for a disease that has long baffled the physician's skill."*

To give it a quantitative measure, I've tracked my BASDAI score against my fasting times. BASDAI is a standard measurement used in rheumatology to judge a patient's level of disease severity. Without fail, fasting always brings down the severity of my disease.

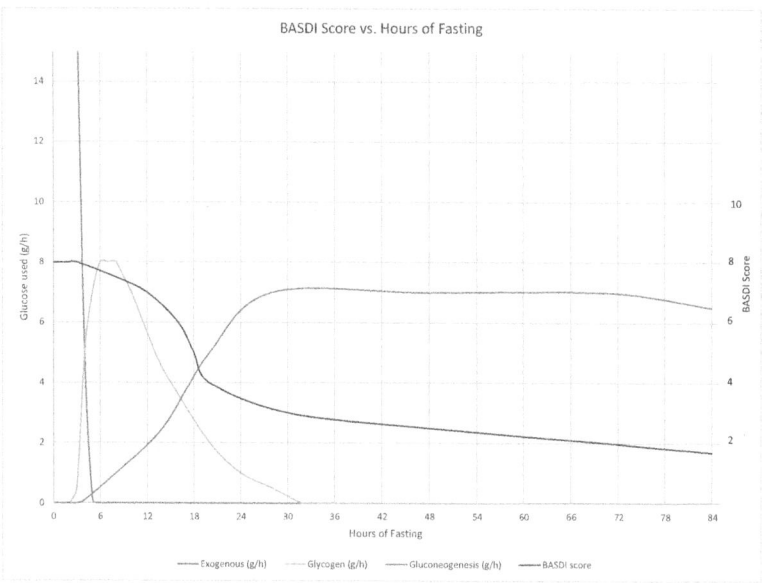

*This chart overlays my personal BASDI Scores during fasting, over the typically established metabolic stages between the postabsorptive state and the near-steady state of prolonged starvation. BASDI scores were consistently improved, markedly around 16–18 hours.*

## Body mass index

When fasting, I used my body mass index (BMI) as a general guide to understand how much I could or should fast. There are a lot of criticisms of the BMI, as it is a very simple metric based on height and weight, so you need to apply this to your own body type and level of athleticism. I found once I accounted for my own level of comfort regarding weight loss and weight gain, it proved to be a good measuring stick in the fasting process. I created upper and lower limits, based on my BMI score, but also considered how I physically felt at these different weights. I always kept my weight in a safe range, never going below 21 on the BMI scale.

**BMI Tracking**

| | | |
|---|---|---|
| Height | 5'10-3/4" | feet,inches |
| Height | 70.75 | inches |
| Weight (empty) | 163 | lbs |
| BMI | 22.9 | |
| Weight (fed) | 170 | lbs |
| BMI | 23.9 | |
| Average BMI | **23.4** | |

| | Score | Weight | Diet Strategy |
|---|---|---|---|
| Underweight | 18.5 | 132 | Gain weight |
| Fasting limit | 20 | 142 | No Fasting at or below this value (based on medical recommendations) |
| | 20.3 | 145 | Average BMI of Hadza Hunter Gatherers |
| Low Energy, weak feeling, BMI Lower target | 21 | 150 | No Fasting at or below this value (based on personal feel, energy levels) |
| BMI target, BSW? | 22 | 157 | Maintenence |
| BMI target, BSW? | 23 | 164 | Fasting ok. Feel no energy loss fasting at this weight |
| Overweight feeling, BMI Upper Target | 24 | 171 | Feel heavier and an actual desier to start fasting at this weight |
| Overweight per BMI | 25 | 178 | Increase fasting |

Also included are the results of some of my fasts, which show the actual, average weight loss per day. As I became more active, I tended toward the upper end of this scale. I feel that the additional weights, Pilates and upper body exercises may have increased muscle mass, so I felt more comfortable and more energetic when I was near the upper end of my "normal" BMI range.

These are the total weight loss results of my seven-day water fast.

# FASTING TO REDUCE INFLAMMATION

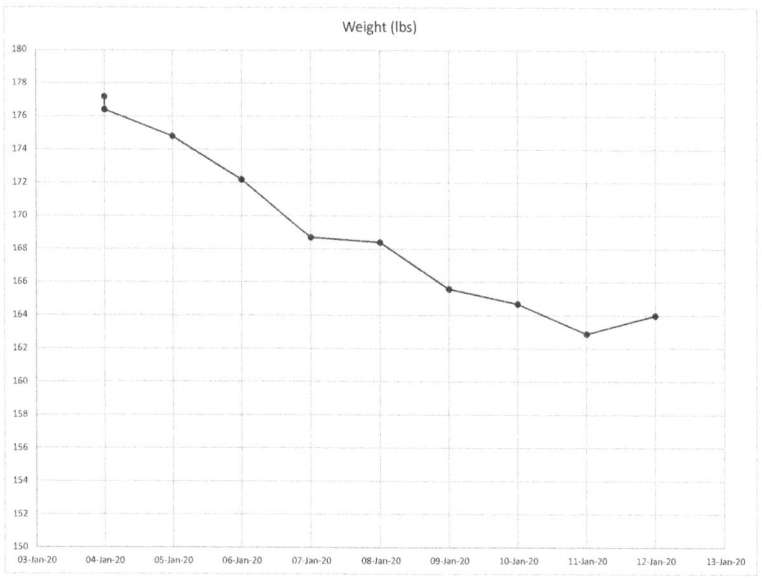

Reduction of body fat over the seven days, from approximately 19.5% to 16.9%, which represents 7.5 lbs of body fat:

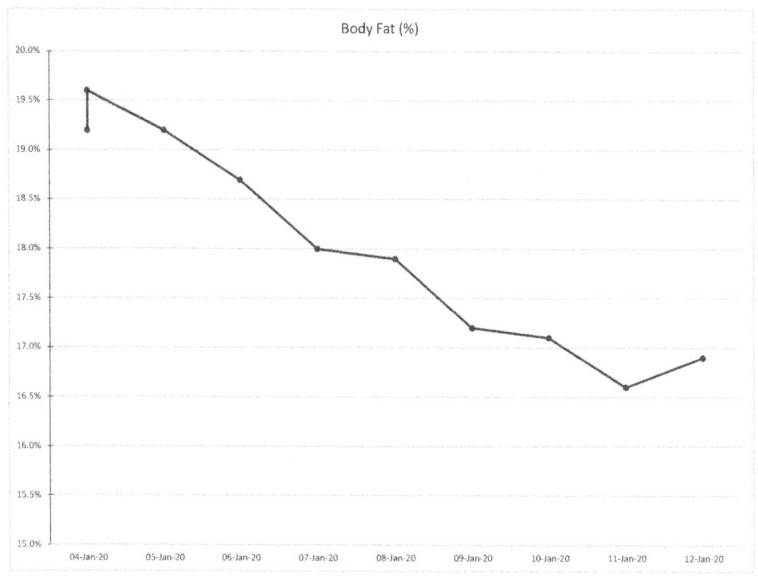

However, notice that while staying active during the water fast, there was virtually no loss in muscle mass, less than 0.5 lbs.

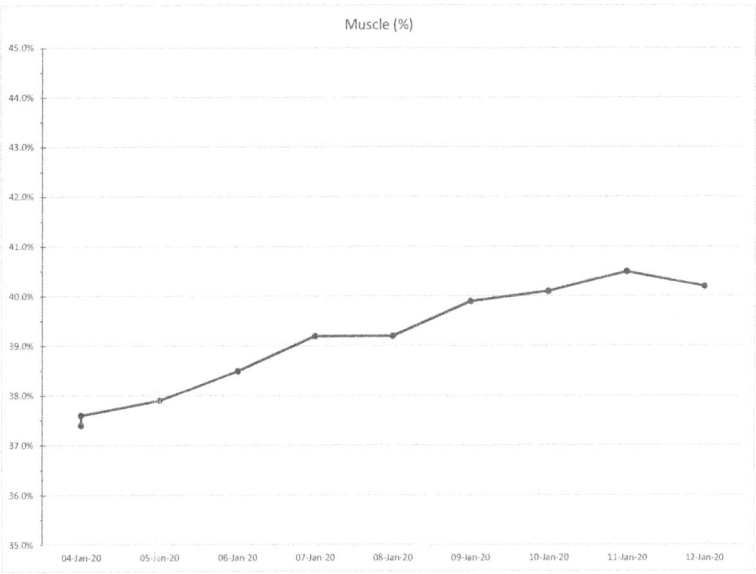

This data was collected using bioelectric impedance analysis. Data points were taken at the same time each day for consistency.

## Refeeding after fasting

Refeeding syndrome describes metabolic disturbances that occur when food is reintroduced when the body is starved, malnourished, or metabolically stressed due to severe illness. Reintroducing food and nutrition activates hormones like insulin, which triggers the body to produce glycogen, fat, and protein in cells. The body pulls minerals into the cells to accomplish this. When this occurs too quickly, before the body has a chance to replenish stores, refeeding syndrome can occur. (Hisham M Mehanna, 2008)

The primary concern is the body's usage of phosphorus, potassium, calcium, and magnesium. If usage occurs too quickly, too little of these minerals are left in the blood. This is what causes the major symptoms of the refeeding syndrome, some of which can be fatal in extreme circumstances.

The first mineral to consider is phosphorus. Very low phosphorus levels in the blood is called hypophosphatemia. If you took a high school biology course, you may remember that phosphorus is used in all cells for energy, by the creation of an adenosine triphosphate (ATP) molecule that contains three phosphorus molecules. So, severe depletion of phosphorus may cause your entire body to "power down." Serum phosphate concentrations below a certain level (0.81 mmol/L) can result muscle weakness, respiratory failure and difficulty breathing, and heart failure.

Magnesium is involved in most enzyme systems in the body and severe depletion can result in cramps, confusion, tremor, tetany and occasionally, seizures, which is classically the pattern known as "Torsades de Pointes." Most magnesium (about 70%) taken orally is not absorbed but excreted unchanged in the feces.

Potassium may also be shifted into cells, leaving dangerously low levels in the blood; this is known as hypokalemia. This too can cause heart rhythm disturbances or even cardiac arrest.

The necessity of minerals is why I try to focus on nutrient-dense natural foods, as listed before, during my feeding periods, since I fast intermittently as well. I think back on the way I used to eat before the onset of my AS, and how many meals and snacks I had that were really just empty calories, with very little nutrition at all. I may as well have skipped those meals entirely for the good of my health.

Insulin stimulates glycogen, fat and protein synthesis, which requires many ions like phosphorus, magnesium, and thiamine. The stores of all these minerals have been depleted during fasting and once refeeding begins, too much phosphorus may be taken out of the blood by the body, leading to excessively low levels.

Therefore, it makes the most sense to start feeding slowly, with low-glycemic index foods that don't raise insulin too quickly or too severely, and foods that contain these four minerals, including thiamine. Half-size meals have worked well for me and given my body a time to adjust.

In my own experience, the problems I've had with refeeding are generally the result of overfeeding too much food, too soon. My fasts have generally been quite short, less than 7 days, so I've not been at risk of any serious mineral depletion. During my longest fast, I've experienced minor swelling in the legs and feet, and I chose to end that particular fast because of it. I was using salt water during my fast, and too much salt seemed to cause increased water retention. Subsequent fasts were done with regular mineral water, and I did not have the same symptoms.

Generally, I found refeeding too quickly or using the wrong foods to cause diarrhea, upset stomach or bloating. After a few tries, this is the formula that has worked best for me:

## Best refeeding foods (organized by nutrient)

For phosphorus: (before any insulin-spiking foods):
- Dark leafy greens
- Swiss cheese (567 mg/100 g)
- Trout (269 mg/100 g), in moderation, high protein
- Egg (191 mg/100 g)
- Herring (89 mg/100 g), in moderation, high protein

- Milk (86 mg/100 ml), not recommended, avoid dairy during refeeding
- Basil (56 mg/100 g)
- Avocado (52 mg/100 g)

For magnesium (for heart considerations as described before):
- Dark leafy greens like spinach (79 mg/100 g)
- Basil (64 mg/100 g)
- Escargot (62% DV), in moderation due to protein
- Flax (98% DV)

For thiamine (B1) (coenzyme in carb metabolism):
- Flax Seeds (1.6 mg/ 100 g)
- Macadamias (1.2 mg/100 g), low carb, low starch, low protein
- Trout (0.43 mg/100 g), caution, high protein
- Salmon (0.3 mg/100 g)
- Egg (.08 mg/100 g)
- Herring (.07 mg/100 g), caution, high protein

For potassium:
- Avocado (485 mg/ 100g)
- Salmon (352 mg/ 100g)
- Spinach (336 mg/100 g)
- Broccoli (184 mg/ 100g)
- Lime (102 mg/ 100g)

For calcium:
- Cheese (721 mg/ 100g)
- Chia seeds (631 mg/ 100g)
- Sardines, canned with bones (382 mg/ 100g)
- Flax (255 mg/ 100g)

For vitamin D:
- Salmon, tuna, mackerel (240 IU – 988 IU/ 100g)
- Egg yolk, one large (25 IU)

For Vitamin B12:
- Mussels (25.4 mcg/ 100g)
- Sardines (9.4 mcg/ 100g)
- Cheese (0.8 mcg/ 100g

For vitamin K:
- Kale (449 mcg/ 100g)
- Parsley (416 mcg/ 100g)
- Spinach (375 mcg/ 100g)

## Recommended meals for refeeding after a fast

By far the number one rule: 50% calorie requirements, and reintroduce foods slowly!

- Foods high in the minerals listed before
- Very low-GI foods and low-carb type foods
- Do not refeed with carbohydrates
- Do not refeed on milk
- Do not start with citrus or fibre

## Order to reintroduce foods

First day

Minerals and hydration first:
- Vegetable juice: dark leafy greens, cucumber, lime, celery
- Vegetable broth: celery, garlic, onion, bell pepper, add fish or chicken bone, ensure it is only a small serving of protein
- Spinach, egg

Second day

Thiamine:
- Egg, seaweed, macadamias
- Trout/herring/sardine
- Avocado (half of fruit to maintain low carbs)

Fats (These are more difficult to digest, although I've experienced no problems myself and they seem beneficial in providing some energy and helping prevent food from passing through the body too quickly. I've tried starting with these foods after a four-day fast with no problems or discomfort.):

- Ghee, butter, mayonnaise, olive oil
- Fatty fish
- Macadamias
- Egg
- Avocado

Proteins (Although in moderation because protein can also increase insulin. I've found protein to give me rosacea after a fast.):

- Fish, egg, cheese, although I have introduced these on my first day of refeeding without any problems

Carbs (These are last as they cause fluid retention.):
- Transition to carbs and fibre with egg, macadamias, flax/chia/hemp
- Vegetable smoothie: kale, spinach, lettuce, sprouts

After transitioning back to the fed state, I've found that this diet seems to match my ideal long-term diet, with a focus on nutrients from vegetables, the majority of my calories from healthy fats, only a moderate amount of protein, and the least emphasis on carbs.

*There is a tendency on the part of the faster to overeat, not alone because he is hungry, but also because he is desirous of regaining his weight. His friends also urge him to eat. Sinclair truly says: "A person at the end of a (long) fast is an agitating sight to his neighbors, and their one impulse is to get a 'square meal' into him as quickly as possible."*

-Fasting Cure - Sinclair

# CHAPTER 7

# ANTI-INFLAMMATORY FOODS AND DIET

Our closest relationship with our surrounding environment is through our air, water and food. The gut has a surface area 40 times larger than the surface area of our skin, so what we eat is incredibly important in determining what we are exposed to in our environment. There are many studies and much research that shows that diet has an impact on AS and other types of arthritis as well. Antigens entering our body such as bacteria, animal proteins, and oils can create an inflammatory response. However, I get the impression that most of the well-established arthritis societies are very conservative in prescribing food as a treatment for arthritis. One reason, is that every individual's bacterial biome is as individual as a fingerprint, meaning everyone will have a different list of foods that benefit them most.

This is why I would recommend anyone conduct an elimination diet as I have, to determine which foods work best for them. For AS, wheat, corn, sugar and lentils are the most common, however, processed meats (and processed foods in general) and to a lesser extent, dairy products, eggs, and many others can be problems, but are more applicable to autoimmune disease in general. Using fasting as a "cleansing" period before trying other foods can make patterns or certain food problems much clearer, clearing arthritis pain and providing a good baseline when reintroducing foods.

## Foods

Despite the recommendation for everyone to conduct their own elimination diet to determine which foods work the best for them, there are many foods that, through studies, we already know will work for most. Therefore, that's the best place to start.

I've been given the advice to get my macro nutrients (fat, protein and carbohydrates) in the correct proportions as a priority, but over the years I feel it's been better to focus on micronutrients as a priority, always making sure to obtain nutrient-dense foods from plant sources first and nutrients from animal sources second. A moderate balance of protein should be achieved and then fill in your calorie requirements with fats.

You don't need much focus on protein, if you're getting the right nutrient-dense foods in, including some fish (which is one of my most recommended foods); your protein intake will take care of itself. Much current research now agrees that we get much more protein than we actually need from diet alone, and extra protein can even be converted to sugar and may contribute to inflammation and a plethora of other health problems. The general recommendation is 0.8 g/kg per day. At my weight, I required about 60 g of protein a day. When I tracked my calorie intake on a daily basis, I would regularly exceed my protein intake without trying. Especially with chicken in my diet, there were days when I could easily double my intake requirement. I'm not a bodybuilder, but I'm moderately muscular and active, train with weights, and protein intake has never been in short supply.

One of the earlier studies I came across indicated that (in rheumatoid arthritis patients) a totally fat-free diet for seven weeks resulted in complete remission of arthritis pain, and a reintroduction of animal fat and protein, and vegetable fats, caused a return of symptoms. (Alan Goldhamer, 1997) However, through my own research and experience, I feel that this fat-free recommendation, or the recommendation to avoid animal products, is so generalized that it misses the true cause, since the study did not consider the type or source of fat. In addition, going truly fat free as a long-term solution is very difficult and definitely not healthy. I will discuss this in more detail later, but very clearly, some fats are anti-inflammatory, and some are inflammatory, and the type of fat we are consuming is important.

As for carbohydrates, they can be kept to a minimum, especially the starches, however, there are a few fruits that I highly recommend as sources of antioxidants.

This is a list of my most recommended foods. Some recommendations are based on studies. In those cases, I provide a reference to the study where I found the information. Some have given me clear benefit, and others I haven't noticed any benefit, but I would like to keep them here in case they help others, as they have reports of being beneficial. In the section "Assessment of treatment effectiveness," I will go into more detail on that foods provided a noticeable benefit in my experience with managing AS. I list them in order of benefit, from greatest to least, in each of their respective food groups.

\* = Did not personally notice clear benefit, but supported by studies
\*\* = Noticeable benefit and strongly supported by studies
XX = Noticeable detriment

## Nutrients – vegetables (all non-root veggies)

- **Fresh* garlic 10–20 g or 6–7 cloves (contains allicin to suppress HLA-B27); also linked to reduced risk of prostate cancer, contains inulin and oligofructose. Increases IL-10 (which represses TNF and other inflammatory cytokines). Promotes *Lactobacillus* and *Bifidobacterium*. Sulfur rich so promotes glutathione production. This can be hard in practice, especially if your significant other doesn't like garlic breath! Marinated or cooked garlic damages the allicin, so it needs to be fresh. Chopping or crushing and combining with other foods is a good option.
- *Broccoli (anti-inflammatory by reducing cytokines and NF-kB, high in antioxidants, vitamin A, melatonin). High in fibre and sulfur. Best raw or lightly steamed.
- *Fermented or raw cabbage (vitamin C and contains proline, which, together with glycine, helps form collagen for joint growth). High in fibre.
- *Zucchini (for pectin, potassium, sodium-potassium combination is anti-inflammatory and flushing, antioxidants, good for eye health).
- *Cauliflower, vitamin C, quercetin, fibre, complete protein, high in a-linolenic acid (ALA) omega-3, low-carb, iron, sulfur, best in raw form. Careful with overconsumption as it has high fermentation potential in the gut.
- *Bok choy (vitamin C, phytonutrient antioxidants, flavaols like quercetin).
- *Celery (flavonoid and polyphenols to reduce inflammation, flavaols like quercetin). Fibre.
- Kale (preferred over chard and spinach, to lower oxalic acid levels and reduce kidney stone risk). High in folate, vitamin A, vitamin E, iron, some protein, and quercetin).

- *Spinach (magnesium, vitamin A, vitamin E, beta carotene, alpha lipoic acid). Fibre, very low-carb, best boiled or cooked to release more iron and minerals from oxalates.
- Raw red onion (quercetin). Green onion for phosphorous, magnesium, vitamin K; onion, for inulin and oligofructose. Again, has high fermentation potential so avoid over consumption.
- Alfalfa or garlic sprouts contain isoflavones which supports DHA and suppresses AA.
- Asparagus (good fibre, iron and antioxidants, quercetin, melatonin, has inulin which supports beneficial lactobacilli and *Bifidobacteria*).
- Mushrooms for niacin (B3, 34% DV/cup, 21.9 mg).

## Nutrients – animals

- *Fish skin (glycine, proline for joint healing, lysine, arginine, healing and immune system function).
- Chicken liver (CoQ10, 11.6 mg/100 g).
- Fish bone (soft bones in canned fish, like sardines and salmon).
- Fish bone broth (use heads, gills removed, try 1–2 hours, try non-oily like sole, snapper, rockfish, or try mackerel, or oily like salmon).
- *Gelatin (glycine, Proline, lysine). 10g/day.
- Chicken-feet broth.

## Fats

- *Fish (Atlantic mackerel, sardines, herring [vitamin D], trout, Anchovy). These are high in omega-3 EPA, DHA (aim for 2.7–5 g/day for three months, minimum). (Lee YH1, 2012) Also high in lysine. Sardines high in selenium. These small fish are typically low in mercury and are therefore safe to eat on a regular basis, and they contain high amounts of omega-3 EPA and DHA. Many are also high in lysine. Herring is also very high in vitamin D. Other fish I recommend are fatty fish like wild salmon, which is also high in the omega-3s and antioxidants. Since the onset of my condition, I've been aiming for 2.7–5 g/day of omega-3s. Plan to obtain this quantity, for three months minimum before you start to see benefits. There are many studies that show omega-3 oils, specifically the EPA and DHA sourced from fish, help reduce inflammation. Omega-3 has also been shown to suppress LTB4 (R I Sperling, Dietary omega-3 polyunsaturated fatty acids inhibit phosphoinositide formation and chemotaxis in neutrophils., 1993) If buying canned fish, try to purchase fish in water and not oil, or choose olive oil above something like safflower or canola oil to limit your omega-6 intake, which has an inflammatory property in the body (AP1., 2002).

- **Black olives or olive oil (oleocanthal from olive oil as anti-inflammatory [50 g = 1/10 ibuprofen] and high omega-9 [monounsaturated], low omega-6 [contains oleocanthal which prevents the production of COX-1 and COX-2], 11:1 omega-6:3 with 1.1 g omega-6 per Tbsp, melatonin, CoQ10 [11.4 mg/100 g]). Strive for 100 g/day (approximately two shots).
- Coconut oil (anti-inflammatory, sterols promote natural steroid hormones including corticosteroids which help control inflammation). MCT oil (part of coconut oil).
- Avocado or avocado oil. Anti-inflammatory omega-9 and vitamin E, but still in moderation due to high omega-6, good fibre.
- Butter/ghee (lactose and casein free, contains conjugated linoleic acid [CLA] to reduce body fat, prevent cancer, butyric acid for inflammation).

- Dark chocolate (cocoa powder, very high in polyphenols to help reduce inflammation, flavonoids, zinc, minerals). Be sure to check sugar content.

## Protein

- Mussels (high in iron, B12 and protein, balanced 6:3 omega, 0.3 g/100 g omega-6), clams, oysters, crab, shrimp, scallops, octopus, nearly any seafood, just watch mercury content.
- Chia (good gamma linolenic acid (GLA) oils, complete protein).
- Flax. Soak/sprout on paper to reduce phytic acid content, if possible, or consume flax oil instead.
- Spirulina could stimulate your immune system and make condition worse. (UC Davis Health, 2000) I've had this on several occasions but not clear of any effect.

## Carbohydrates (grains/nuts/seeds, other)

- Macadamia nuts. Low-carb content and lowest omega-6 (.7g/100g) content. Good iron and magnesium, fibre. High calorie. Low-resistant starch (RS) 1g/100g, iodine tested ok.
- Broccoli, for fibre which contributes to butyrate production in the gut and reduced gut inflammation.

## Carbohydrates (fruit) (generally all fruit are ok but in moderation due to sugar)

- **Goldenberries (target COX-2, decrease TNFα, IL-6, increases HO-1 antioxidant enzyme and Nrf2 to defend against tissue damage, lowers IL-9, decreases MCP-1 and ERK signalling to lower inflammation, IL-6, IL-10, IL-1B). These little berries seem to be very effective and almost always feel better the next day so I highly recommend them.

- **Pomegranate (TNF expression is unregulated by punicic acid in seed, blocks COX enzyme activity which regulates production of prostaglandins, is high in flavonoids, hydrobenzoic acid, shown to be anti-prostate cancer, high antioxidants, melatonin). In moderation, high in sugar.
- *Pineapple (contains bromelain to reduce prostaglandins, works together with quercetin).
- Blueberry and strawberry (anthocyanins are anti-inflammatory).
- Blueberries (resveratrol, again more for colitis) and for quercetin, raspberries (high in fibre).
- Black current (very high in vitamin C).
- Berries (dark red fruits, for flavonoids).
- Apple (peel) (high in ursolic acid, like rosemary, source of Quercetin, COX2 inhibitor, IL-17 inhibitor).

## Supplements

In general, foods are safer than supplements, as it is much more difficult to get too much of any particular nutrient from food than it is from taking supplements. Nutrients in foods obviously undergo less processing than synthetic supplements. Despite this, some supplements are beneficial for managing arthritis.

- **Omega-3 EPA and DHA. The benefits from fish oils are long term and this supplement needs to be taken every day, with results gradually observable over a 4+ week duration, but many studies show this type of fat is anti-inflammatory.
- Glycine (2–20 g/day, try for 10 g/d, can be used safely in high doses of 15–60 g/day (by my weight, 30–60 g/day recommended) although 25 g is considered a conservative max dose. Source instead from a good quality gelatin (about 33% glycine) if possible.

- **Gelatin (including bone broth, meat, poultry, eggs, spinach, kale, banana). TNF antagonist and builds connective tissue with proline, promotes restful sleep and fights fatigue caused by anemia.
- **Cat's claw (major TNF antagonist (20–60 mg/d in capsule)).
- *Ferrous Gluconate (iron, 78 mg/d). Recommended if you are managing anemia due to low iron. Remember to avoid combining iron supplements with coffee, tea or calcium in the same meal, and take with vitamin on an empty stomach, if possible, to help absorption.
- *Oregano oil to kill *Klebsiella*. Personally, I had difficulty correlating this specifically to changes in pain, and studies only show its efficacy in vitro, but it may be worth a try.
- Curcumin. I did not notice any benefit from curcumin but there are studies that this is beneficial when taken with pepper.
- *Green tea (high in flavonoids, reduces cytokines. Not with a meal, since tannins can inhibit iron absorption and contribute to anemia).
- *Rosemary tea (consume 4-6 g/d or .1–1 ml of essential oil, ursolic acid inhibits IL-17, in moderation, since may also cause DNA damage).
- *White willow bark.
- Vitamin D (source from herring).
- Vitamin B6 (pyridoxine).
- Vitamin E (alpha and gamma tocopherol, supplementation resulted in relief of pain) (Bioconcepts, 2018).
- *Vitamin C (limit to one gram per day if taking consistently) and other antioxidants like vitamin E, beta carotene, coenzyme Q10, catalase, superoxide dismutase, selenium and zinc. Reduce and get more from diet (bell peppers, broccoli, cabbage), and note that more than one gram per

day may increase risk of kidney stones. (Brianna Elliot, 2017)
- Mustard. Increases IL-10.
- Inulin (fibre). This is a fructan and is consistent with FODMAP issues, however, this tested in my diet with no problems (August 9, 2018), but also with no added benefit, except to avoid constipation during fasting.
- *Pycnogenol (Maritime pine bark).
- Field Horsetail, known by its scientific name *Equisetum arvense*, shows very strong antimicrobial activity against *Klebsiella pneumoniae* among others, including *Candida albicans* (A. Pallag, 2018). Harvested in May/June, when the flavonoid content in the plant is highest.
- Grapefruit seed extract. Free radical TNFα and NF-kB lowering.

## Probiotics

Probiotics are microorganisms commonly found in certain foods that are believed to have beneficial health effects. In AS, they are believed to have benefit as healthy bacteria that colonize the intestinal tract and help to crowd out *Klebsiella*.

Not everyone agrees in the effectiveness of probiotics. In a recent BBC article, probiotics were labelled "quite useless." *"And in that sense just buying probiotics at the supermarket without any tailoring, without any adjustment to the host, at least in part of the population, is quite useless."* (Gallagher J., 2018)

One point this article does make, however, is that the good bacteria need to be continually supplied, or a person's microbiome will return to its usual state.

However, in this book we are not dealing with the healthy, general population. We are discussing people with AS. Therefore, I believe it's more valuable to look at studies that assess probiotics specifically in the light of AS, including *Lactobacillus rhamnosus* GG.

What is clear is that these microbes profoundly influence the immune response.

> *"Accordingly an HLA B27 positive rat that normally develops colitis, skin lesions, and arthropathy remains generally healthy in a germ free environment [26] and several murine models of colitis are also cured by a germ free environment [27]."*

> *"Colitis in the HLA B27 transgenic rat model can be effectively prevented with antibiotics, and this benefit can be maintained if the rat is colonized with Lactobacillus Rhamnosus but not by Lactobacillus plantarum [31]. In contrast, Lactobacillus Bifidus will induce arthritis in germ free mice which lack the IL-1 receptor antagonist [32]."* (James T. Rosenbaum, 2011)

*Lactobacillus rhamnosus*, in particular, seems to be a beneficial little microbe, providing influence on our brains by reducing anxiety, and we know there is a link between anxiety and increased arthritis pain. (Javier A. Bravo, 2011) Interestingly, when I was on week-long work trip, I tried to eat well and keep my omega-3s up and my omega-6s and resistant starches down. The one thing I didn't do was keep my healthy probiotics up. When I returned from my trip and reintroduced kefir and kombucha, my lower-back pain was markedly reduced, even though the rest of my diet did not change. The theory behind this is that the good bacteria will "crowd out" the bad, *Klebsiella* bacteria. The correlation is not as strong as some of the other factors in this book, but it is definitely there, and something I would recommend for someone with arthritis and especially AS. *Lactobacillus rhamnosus* GG is a probiotic commonly found in milk kefir and drinkable yogurts and is recommended to prevent traveller's diarrhea. You are supposed to start taking it two or three days before you travel and keep taking it daily throughout the trip. (Cerner Multum, Inc., 2018) Interestingly, my AS started with diarrhea symptoms during travel. I now make and consume my own kefir daily.

*Lactobacillus casei* (DN-114 001) is a strain found in some dairy products like yogurt, which in studies has been shown to significantly decrease secretion of the pro-inflammatory cytokines TNFα and IL-6, and appeared to inhibit the COX-2 pathway and NF-kB. (Healing Arthritis, Susan Blum, P.97)

*Lactobacillus acidophilus* (CL1285) plus *Lactobicillus casei* (Lbc80r) is shown in animal studies to protect against damage to the joints, which is believed to result from systemic inflammation.

From my personal experience, there is correlation between gut activity and arthritis pain. Using these probiotics has shown to provide benefit.

## Foods in moderation

Some foods appear to have positive and negative benefits. There may be anti-inflammatory properties that can benefit arthritis in general, but they may also cause problems in higher amounts due to starch if you have AS. I've listed some of these foods here.

## Vegetables

- Peppers (for vitamin C, vitamin A and quercetin). Recommended together with chia. In moderation due to lectin content if you find it gives you stomach issues.
- *Ginger, bactericidal against *Klebsiella* (in vitro) and for inflammation in colitis. Caution, iodine tested black, and my personal log shows a weak association with foot pain.
- Brussels spouts (contain glucosinolates [glucobrassicin] and vitamin K and ALA omega-3 to reduce inflammatory cytokines). Generally a great food but if you have AS, exercise caution, iodine tested black indicating starch.
- Pumpkin, (starch=1.7 g/100 g [calculated], mostly monosaccharides). Tested ok in diet, higher quantities seem to cause mild reaction in feet.
- Winter squash soup. Ok based on testing.
- Spaghetti squash (starch=2.7 g/100 g [calculated]).Tested ok in diet.
- Carrots (1 g RS). Keep to very small quantities.
- Tomato (best cooked to reduce lectin content, high in trans lycopene, although cis lycopene in *Chlorella marina* is more effective).
- Eggplant, in moderation due to lectin.

## Oils

- Walnut (ALA omega-3, GLA omega-6). I had large quantities on several occasions with no effect. Exercise caution; after a few days of walnuts, my neck and back felt worse, and my personal decision was to stay clear and focus on other foods.
- Rapeseed, canola, walnuts, chia and hemp (shouldn't cause harm, omega-6 content is GLA).

- Hemp. Ok per iodide testing, omega-6 content is GLA (not AA) so this is anti-inflammatory. Good vegetable protein. In moderation due to LA omega-6.

## *Proteins*

- *Kefir (for probiotic). Limit to 250 ml/day to limit bloating. Casein (the protein in milk) is a potential issue in RA but should not be a problem in AS, unless you have specific allergies. Casein stimulates prostate cancer cell growth but is also antimutagenic and can lower colon cancer risk. Feeding good bacteria is just as important as limiting *Klebsiella* and I always felt fine consuming it, so I'm keeping it on my recommended list. Antigens from the gut microbiota, rather than food, have been suggested as being more involved in AS, which does fit the *Klebsiella* theory. Full-fat dairy also contains butyrate, which reduces colon inflammation.
- *Cheese, Jarlsberg, Swiss (high protein, good cholesterol, zero lactose, zero carb, zero sugar) and is anti-inflammatory, omega-6 is low (0.6 g/100 g). Dry curd cottage cheese (to avoid lactose), very low omega-6, any non-processed cheese should be fine. Aged cheeses are lower in lactose. Otherwise, I've never seen any adverse reactions to large amounts of cheese. Some may choose to limit dairy due to lectin content. I may have noticed an improvement away from dairy when camping, but it was a one-off occurrence and I wasn't able to observe the correlation a second time.
- Lean beef, generally less AA or LA omega-6 than egg or chicken.
- Chicken or other meats, lean, no skin, no fat, no processing. (Processed meats such as bacon, ham, sausages or salami are not quite as healthy as unprocessed meats and should be eaten in moderation.) Keep to a minimum. Free range

(not grain fed), lean cuts like skinless chicken breast seem ok, but don't need to over-consume protein. (Dawn, 2012) Watch omega-6 content. Watch out for high omega-6 from animal fat.
- Eggs (Eggs from chickens with flax in their diet are closer to 1:1 and have ALA omega-3.) Otherwise, in moderation due to AA content (.4 g/egg, .6 g total omega-6). Whites should be cooked, which actually increases protein availability (as opposed to meat).

## Nuts, Grains, carbs

- Chia, in moderation. When you eat high-phytate foods with most of your meals, mineral deficiencies may develop over time.
- Flax or flax oil (good omega-3 [ALA], moderate omega-6). Total starch is approximately 0.4g/100g, iodine tested brown. Diet tested ok. Daily flax seems to feel good. In moderation, too much can cause gassiness which seemed to be associated with evening pain. Also, flax for men should be in moderation due to phytoestrogen content, However, flaxseed oil does not have these phytoestrogens.
- Quick bread, made with flax/chia/kefir/egg/baking soda. A few days in a row I felt general puffiness in my neck, hands and feet (feels like water retention) before bed and the next morning. Also, significant bloating before bed. Kefir and baking soda seem to be a bad mix. Bread works fine when I leave out the baking soda.
- Refined white flour. The brand I use contains added amylase. If I make some homemade bread with this flour, I have no reaction when eaten in moderation (maximum two slices). Amylose content may be low, or the added amylase enzyme may help break down the starch before it reaches the intestine. While refined white flour isn't the healthiest

option, I have to note that I've found it tolerable, and it stands out among other starches that give me a reaction. Calculated total starch is 70 g/100 g, which is very high, but how much of this is amylopectin? How much does the added amylase help? It turns black when tested with iodine, but the amylose portion must be low because it does not illicit an inflammatory reaction.
- Amaranth flour tested ok in moderate quantities in bread. Caution though because this contains moderate amounts of starch, I calculated approximately 16.9 g/100 g.
- Glutinous rice flour (almost 100% amylopectin, very low resistant starch amylose). There must be some amylose still in the rice, as it iodine tested black. Calculated total starch quantity is 19.9 g/100 g, but again this is mostly amylopectin. Consuming a moderate to large serving will make me warm, high energy, even flushed in the face due to its high glycemic index. However, like the refined white flour, this has not caused an inflammatory response in moderate quantities.
- Walnuts (omega-6:3 is 4.2:1, but total omega-3 is 10.6 g/oz), tested brown, tested ok in diet, may be beneficial.
- Hazelnuts are moderately low omega-6, RS is 2.7 g/100 g.
- Baking soda (don't use baking powder since it contains corn starch).
- Raw almonds, soaked for 8 hours. Almonds (1:0 but good vitamin E) (12 g total omega-6), and zero RS. Almond milk and matcha lattes with almond milk made without the skin both test ok. Almonds are anti-inflammatory in diet studies: (Liu JF1, 2013). I would recommend eating in moderation due to omega-6 content.

## ANTI-INFLAMMATORY FOODS AND DIET

*Fruit*

- Minimal high-sugar fruits like bananas, oranges, grapes, mangoes or pineapples, at least if your symptoms are severe. Apples and pears are pretty sugary too.
- *Grapes have very low disaccharides and moderate to low GL, good for an energy boost when fatigued, and also good source of resveratrol and reduce NF-kB.
- Raisins are ok.
- Cherries, tangerines.
- All other fruit should be ok in moderation except bananas.

*Others*

- *Honey is bactericidal against *Klebsiella*, in moderation due to sugar content.
- Dark chocolate (85–90% cacao) check sugar and carb content, no starch (contain flavonoids, which inhibit initial stage of inflammatory cascade). No milk chocolate, chocolate with sugar added or emulsified chocolate.
- Caffeine (caffeine blocks adenosine receptors, and adenosine [naturally occurring in the body] is believed to be an anti-inflammatory agent).
- Coffee? Coffee drinkers had an average of 28% higher TNF, but maybe people with high TNF are tired, so they're more likely to drink coffee. Contains polyphenols that block iron absorption (wait 30 minutes after a meal to avoid interference with iron absorption).
- Dairy, watch omega-6 AA content and sugar (lactose) content. Casein (whey protein products) seems not to be a problem, and saturated fats from dairy (cheese especially soft cheese, dairy) all tested ok. Large quantities of soft cheese (paneer) with no negative effect. Ricotta, cottage cheese, I had in large quantities (consumed together with

big plate of veggies) with no effect. Suspect I had a reaction to buttermilk (possibly due to a larger quantity of lactose) but I was not able to illicit the same response on a second occasion. However, it is noted that substituting saturated fats with mono or polyunsaturated fats eliminates the pro-inflammatory activity of lipopolysaccharides, which prevents an entire cascade of inflammatory activity, including the expression of NF-kB, TNF-a, IL-1, IL-6 and IL-8. (Fritsche, 2015)
- I can tolerate a little bit of sugary food, on a full stomach or with lots of fat, I believe, because it helps keep the insulin spike low. However, it is best to avoid sugary foods (refined and added sugars) all together. Now that I've eliminated sugary food from my diet for quite some time, having sweets will cause me to flush in the face, as if I've just had some liquor.
- Dates or dried fruits in general. No reaction but high in sugar so eat in moderation.

## Foods (and habits) to avoid:

### Overeating

> *"Excessive energy intake promotes inflammation"*
> *(Mark P. Mattson, 2014)*

- XX Undigested carbs are caused by overeating. This might be why I have an unexplained flare after a big meal of foods that are otherwise safe.
- Undigested proteins (primarily from cooked animal proteins) are known to cause inflammation. Excessive protein consumption, especially in a short amount of time, is known to spike insulin and is inflammatory. I have experienced this sort of redness, brain-fog, and very visible

rosacea after protein on many occasions, especially after an intermittent fast.

## Inflammatory oils

The strategy here is to reduce certain oils and fats that promote inflammation through the AA inflammatory pathway. Foods listed here are high in AA and LA omega-6 oils.

- Omega-6 foods, especially nuts and animal fats. Limit omega-6 to 3 g/day.
- XX Oils (peanuts, corn, safflower, sunflower, cottonseed, palm, soy, sesame), excess LA type omega-6 (grapeseed oil, margarine, dressings or spreads based on these oils). Make fish your main protein. Note: despite their bad name, I don't believe all margarines are as bad as they used to be. Many use a moderately healthy blend of canola oil and other oils like avocado or even olive, giving it a reasonable omega-6:3 balance. Read the label to be sure.
- Pecans (20.9:1, total omega-6 is 5.777 g/oz) tested brown, pine nuts, brazil nuts. Avoid due to high LA omega-6.
- Seeds like poppy, sesame, sunflower (LA omega-6).
- Fried foods (high in omega-6 and high temperature causes cancer).
- Trans fats (fried foods, fast food, donuts, cookies, baked goods, margarine) (partially hydrogenated oils).
- Processed or deep-fried poultry (chicken, duck, turkey, high in omega-6). Turkey and chicken sausage (in processed form) have been a problem. Lean, free range chicken breast have, for me, tested ok, or dark meats with minimal animal fat.

## *Synthetics*

- "Modified" ingredients, like modified milk ingredients. As a general rule-of-thumb, anything modified or processed tends to have an inflammatory response in the body.
- XX Processed foods, dietary synthetic emulsifiers or food additives like carrageenan, polysorbate 80 and carboxymethylcellulose CMC. There is evidence in animal studies that these compounds *"induce histopathological features that are typical of IBD while altering the microbiome, disrupting the intestinal epithelial barrier, inhibiting proteins that provide protection against microorganisms, and stimulating the elaboration of pro-inflammatory cytokines".* (J.V. Martino, 2017) They can promote colorectal inflammation and cancer, and include products like mayonnaise, peanut butter, ice cream, puddings, sauces, gum, gelatin products that would naturally separate over time, but also cake, soft drinks, and artificial sweeteners which are bad for gut flora. In fact, foods like zucchini have edible coatings applied to preserve freshness that also contain CMC. Organic foods would be beneficial here to reduce gut inflammation.
- XX Packaged cereals, as they are both typically high in starches and food additives.
- XX Nitrates? Likely this was the cause with chicken sausage (dark meat, charred on the BBQ) that caused major flare-up in feet. I'm finding some sausage and deli meats contain starch, so this may be the true cause. Meats with nitrates but no starch are testing ok.
- Meats cooked at high temperatures, red meat and poultry. (R. Horwitz, 2010)
- XX MSG ("flavoured" foods, chicken broth, noodles, Chinese/Korean takeout, likely the sauce in this case), aspartame.
- Alcohol.

- Smoked meats are associated with increased risk of cancers due to polycyclic aromatic hydrocarbons from wood smoke, increased risk of stomach infection such as *E.coli* (a Gram-negative bacteria like *Klebsiella*) and diarrhea and stomach pain. This is a relatively weak link to AS, but an increased risk of infection may put you at higher risk of AS flares.
- Most major brand chocolates, because they often contain polyglycerol polyricinoleate, an emulsifier. It is generally recognized as safe, but there are other common emulsifiers that are considered inflammatory to the gut. I've noticed some reaction to these chocolates, but the correlation was weak and may have also been due to the sugar content.

## *Sugars*

- Sugar, ingredients ending in -ose (primarily added sugar like sucrose) disrupt insulin, which is connected to hormone activity that affects flares (It triggers the release of inflammatory messengers called cytokines; fructose has the same effect but eating whole fruit [not fruit juice] should temper the dosage.)
- Low-fat dairy products that are traditionally high sugar (cream, yogurt, ice cream).
- Lactose. Of course, if you are lactose intolerant, this is automatically out of your diet, but even for those tolerant of lactose it should be in moderation, as the body converts this to sugar. For me, the problem was with buttermilk, which is very high in lactose. A full cup of buttermilk seemed to set off a flare-up. Also, possibly lactose in cheese triggers flare-up, but this seems to only occur in very high quantities. Good quality cheeses like Swiss that are zero or near-zero in sugar/carb content are no problem.
- High-glycemic index foods, especially white flour.

## Foods that feed Klebsiella

If you have AS, avoid starchy foods, period. There are better tasting foods out there anyway—you just need to know where to look.

- XX Amylose. This type comes from potatoes, corn and starchy fruits such as bananas. Simple carbs: fructose, glucose and apparently sucrose is ok, but limit this. (OK fibres: lignin, cellulose, some hemicellulose, chitin [only weakly]). Should be low RS, typically high-GI grains.
- XX Starchy foods, especially high-amylose foods like lentils, bread, especially whole-grain bread, corn, potatoes, white flour (although some white flour with amylase enzyme may be tolerated), white rice (although glutenous white rice may be tolerated as it is almost entirely amylopectin), white potatoes, most cereals, gluten (wheat, rye, barley and *bran*!), peas, parsnips, squash (such as butternut or acorn, except zucchini and spaghetti), yams, root vegetables, sweet potatoes, taro, cassava radish, beetroot, celeriac, corn, arrowroot, and tapioca.
- XX Modified (corn) starch may be used in low-fat dairy products, pizza toppings, mac and cheese, and lasagna (generally as a fat substitute or thickener).
- XX Deli meats can often have corn starch added. Always read the ingredients listing. Not only is there the potential for the starch to cause problems through the gut, but modified starch is often treated with sodium or potassium hydroxide, potent free radicals, making it doubly likely to cause an arthritis flare. Meat (and meat alone, since I was already avoiding bread) from the deli caused me very clear reactions on two occasions. These meats have given me some of the sharpest reactions in the form of neck and back pain and fatigue, probably since they contained starch, MSG, nitrates and preservatives hitting me all at once.

## ANTI-INFLAMMATORY FOODS AND DIET

- XX Added starch powders, used as a thickener for sauces. Assume all restaurant sauces and non-oil dressings like BBQ, ranch, gravy, pie filling and soup contain it. (Corn starch, potato starch, sweet potato starch, wheat starch, oat starch, tapioca starch, kudzu root starch, arrowroot starch, water chestnut starch or sago starch.)
- XX Baking powder. Exercise caution as some brands have added corn starch.
- Cyclodextrin, used as an emulsifying fibre in mayonnaise, and whipping aids used in desserts and confectioneries.
- Some papers report amylopectin is converted into "limit dextrin," which is also indigestible and is a problem with *Klebsiella*, but reports state glutinous rice flour (amylopectin) is tolerated. In my experience, amylopectin has not caused an inflammatory response on its own.
- Grains, including whole-grain bread, rye bread or pumpernickel (low GL but high RS), wheat, bran, barley, rye, oats, rice, malt, maize, quinoa, buckwheat, spelt, bulgur, couscous, corn, semolina, sorghum, polenta, millet, and etc.
- XX Beans/lentils, including red beans, kidney, pinto (in moderation, this is high RS), and peanut (high in omega-6).
- Seeds like poppy seed, sunflower seeds, sesame seeds, pumpkin and pumpkin seeds.
- XX Nuts. Cashews (higher in omega-6) have repeatedly been shown to contribute to flare-up. It seems high RS is the cause (RS is 12.9, raw cashews 23 g/100 g). Peanut butter. Some brands test black with iodine more readily than others.
- Edamame, for starch content.
- Additives such as microcrystalline cellulose, pregelatinized starch, croscarmellose sodium, colloidal silicon dioxide, ascorbyl palmitate, dextrin, and dextrose.

- XX Gelatinized starches, like gravies, soups, custards, and instant desserts.
- Green/yellow banana (in moderation, RS is .3/100 g). Iodine tested black. For banana with lower starch, consume only very ripe, with black spots or nearly all black skin.
- Sour cream (store-bought brands often have corn starch added, so making your own without starch would be fine, if you tolerate dairy).
- XX Sushi (California rolls) with sauce often have corn starch added; I had a clear reaction to a spicy sashimi sauce that iodine tested black. The rice used is normally sticky rice and very low in amylose. Eating clean sushi or sashimi without any sauce has been ok, causing no reaction.
- XX Cereal. Packaged cereals in general are made from rice ingredients. I tried a bowl full with kefir and was hoping it would act as a prebiotic if taken with a healthy probiotic (kefir) but it still gave me a flare-up. Cereals with corn ingredients gave me a major foot flare-up.

**Nutritional labels**

What's in a nutrition label? It contains a lot of useful information that can help you make healthy eating decisions. The lesser-known fact: what's not on the label also tells you a lot, but it takes a bit of decoding, and you need to look at the ingredients list to understand what's missing.

We will be talking about nutrition labels in Canada, as the legal requirements are different in the United States, although very similar. All major food companies introduced the current nutrition label on packaged foods in 2005. The main information includes calories and 13 nutrients: fat, saturated fat, trans fat, cholesterol, sodium, carbohydrate, fibre, sugars, protein, vitamin A, vitamin C, calcium and iron.

Start with the serving size. You might decide to indulge in a chocolate bar. You've worked hard and it's been a good day. Fat and sugar content is a bit high but not too bad . . . but wait, that's only for three squares! At that rate, this chocolate bar will last as a dessert for four days! My advice would be to stick to the recommended serving size. How much you eat is just as important as what you eat (which is just as important as when you eat, but that's another discussion).

Consider the calories. Also, consider the source of the calories. Different macronutrients have different calorie densities. A gram of fat has about nine calories. A gram of carbohydrates or proteins has about four calories. Of course, this doesn't mean you should avoid fat so you can eat double the carbs and protein. The right type of fat is good for you! Fat in your meal also increases satiety and reduces hunger. Not all carbs are equal either, as easily digested carbs will breakdown into sugar more quickly, spike your blood sugar and insulin levels, and prompt your body to store those extra calories as fat.

The % Daily Value puts nutrients on a scale from 0% to 100%. This scale tells you if there is a little or a lot of a nutrient in one serving of a packaged food. In general, 5% DV or less is a little, and 15% DV or more is a lot.

Total fat calculation:

Often, a label will include total fat, saturated fat and trans fat. Sometimes it will go into more detail and list the contents of other fats as well. The total fat is always a sum of all fats in the food. So, a food label with 8 g of total fat, 1 g of saturated fat, and 0 g of trans fat, means there are 7 g of fat not shown in the total (8 − 1 − 0 = 7). What type of fat? This is where you need to look at the ingredients list and research your food. If one of the main ingredients are chia seeds, you can rest assured that the majority of the fat is anti-inflammatory omega-3 fats, and fewer inflammatory omega-6 fats, since the omega-3:6 ratio in chia is 3:1. Your body needs omega-6 as well, but we generally get way too much omega-6 in the standard American diet.

Total carbs calculation:

Total carbohydrates works the same way. Total carbohydrates listed is the sum of dietary fibre, plus sugars (yes, sugars are carbs) with the remainder of the carbs not shown on the label coming from starches. For example, a label with 37 g of total carbs, with 4 g of fibre and 1 g of sugar, means the food will have 32 g of starch (37 - 4 - 1 = 32). What type of starch? Again, this is where you will need to refer to the ingredients list and research your foods. Using chia as an example again, the majority of chia will be resistant starch, which can feed the healthy bacteria in your gut and act as a prebiotic. The opposite end of the spectrum is something like white rice, which contains a lot of rapidly digestible starch which your body easily breaks down into sugars.

Speaking of sugars, not all sugars are created (or packaged) equally. Naturally occurring sugars, like fructose and glucose, when in their natural packaging (i.e., a piece of fruit) contain enough fibre, and low enough sugars per serving, to be healthy. This is why a sweet and juicy, yet fiberous, portion of watermelon has a glycemic load of only 4, while a white plain bagel can have a glycemic load of 25. Your body is getting a much bigger sugar rush from the rapidly digestible starch in the bagel, which your body converts to sugar. Even sweet, sugary dried dates, with a glycemic load of 18, pack less of a sugar punch than a plain bagel.

## Nutritional claims

What do nutrition claims really mean? If there is a nutrition claim on the label, it must meet a certain legal requirement to be there. There are many, including a long list of terms that indicate what's in the food (for example, processed cheese, or pasteurized process cheese food (PPCF) is only required to contain a minimum of 51% real cheese). Here are some common food claims:

### Source of fibre

"Source of fibre" means the food contains at least 2 g of fibre in the amount of food specified in the Nutrition Facts table. "High source of fibre" means at least 4 g of fibre, and "Very high source of fibre" is at least 6 g of fibre.

### Low fat

"Low fat" means that the food contains no more than 3 g of fat in the amount of food specified in the Nutrition Facts table.

### Cholesterol-free

The claim "cholesterol-free" means that the product has a very small amount (less than 2 mg of cholesterol in the amount of food specified in the Nutrition Facts table) and it is also low in saturated fat and trans fat.

### Sodium-free

A "sodium-free" claim means the amount of food specified in the Nutrition Facts table contains less than 5 mg of sodium.

## Reduced in calories

"Reduced in calories" has at least 25% less energy (calories) than the food it is being compared to. Most of the time, it's being compared to the regular version of that food.

## Light

The term "light" is allowed only on foods that are either "reduced in fat" or "reduced in energy" (calories). "Light" can also be used to describe sensory characteristics of a food, for example, light tasting or light coloured.

## Polyunsaturated fats

The type of fat we have in our diet has been shown to have an impact on the inflammatory processes occurring in the body. We can't do without fat entirely, and society is starting to realize that a good amount of fat in our diet is healthy. When unhealthy fats are consumed, health problems can ensue, and when quantities are too high, combined with a high-carbohydrate diet, it leads to fat accumulation and its associated problems (since both fat and carbs in the diet will lead the body to store the fat, and burn the carbs first). Some fats are even considered essential, such as fats that our body can't synthesize from other compounds.

Mono and poly unsaturated fats are fats that do not have double carbon bonds throughout their molecule, so they are not "saturated" with hydrogen. The length of the carbon chain, the number of double bonds, and the location of the first bond are generally used to classify fats, and the different structure has a major impact on how the body uses the fat.

## Monounsaturated fats

Monounsaturated fats are the best and healthiest fats to add to your diet. Omega-7, called palmitoleic acid, is a 16-molecule-long carbon chain with one double bond at the seventh carbon location (annotated as 16:1 (n-7)), hence it is an omega-"7." This is naturally found in macadamia nuts and is regarded as a healthy, anti-inflammatory oil. I have been able to consume large quantities (much too large, given my love for macadamias) with no inflammatory reactions. Omega-9 (18:1 (n-9)) is called oleic acid, its name being derived from its most abundant source, olives. It's common in olive oil and avocado, and also in high concentrations in pecan, canola, macadamia, high-oleic sunflower oil and flax. Like omega-7, omega-9 is considered healthy and anti-inflammatory. I feel benefit from consuming olive oil in my diet especially, typically 50 g/day is recommended, as it also contains oleocanthal, which has been shown to have the same anti-inflammatory effect as 1/10 of an ibuprofen. It works by preventing the production of the COX-1 and COX-2 prostaglandins.

## Polyunsaturated fats

### Omega-3s

As an arthritis sufferer, the omega-3s EPA and DHA are a must. There are many studies that show these oils are anti-inflammatory, and I am convinced that they are, through my own experience. EPA is a 20:5 (n-3) chain and DHA is a 22:6 (n-3) chain. EPA is non-essential, since the body can produce it from another polyunsaturated fat, ALA; however, the body is inefficient at this process and for AS sufferers, I feel EPA in the diet is a must. It can be obtained through small cold-water fish like herring and sardines, or fatty cold-water fish like salmon.

a-Linolenic acid (ALA) is an omega-3 that is also a healthy anti-inflammatory, but studies show that its anti-inflammatory effects are more focused on the colon. Also beneficial for an AS sufferer, since colon issues are a common comorbidity. The benefit from this omega-3 ends up being less direct than EPA and DHA, but nevertheless, good for you. As already mentioned, the body can also convert ALA into EPA, but not very effectively, so it's still a benefit to obtain EPA in the diet. ALA can be found in chia, flax, fish, hemp hearts (10 g/100 g) and walnuts (2 g/100 g).

LTB4 is a naturally occurring chemical in the body that can cause chronic inflammation (AM1., 2009). Fortunately, through diet, it has been shown that omega-3 oils EPA and DHA, naturally sourced from fish, can suppress LTB4 (R I Sperling, Dietary omega-3 polyunsaturated fatty acids inhibit phosphoinositide formation and chemotaxis in neutrophils., 1993). The quantities of omega-3 in the study are 15 g/day which is quite high—most will recommend no more than 5 g/day on a regular basis—but 15 g/day has been proven to be safe for a limited period of time. Diet plays a huge role when it comes to chronic inflammation in the body. As mentioned, it has been shown that a diet high in fish oil decreases the production of LTB4.

## *Omega-6s*

Much of the discussion around omega-3 and omega-6 these days simplifies the matter to "omega-3s good, omega-6s bad", although this is far from the truth. It is true that the standard American diet (SAD) provides too much omega-6 (most nutritionists will agree that the omega-6:3 ratio should be 4:1 or 1:1, compared to the 25:1 ratio more typically provided with the SAD). We can definitely reduce our omega-6 intake, since it competes with our omega-3 absorption in the body, however some omega-6 is good for you;

some is essential, meaning it is required by the body and the body cannot produce it on its own, and some we can do without.

Conjugated linoleic acid (CLA) is an omega-6, but acts more like an omega-3 in the body. It can be found in butter and ghee. It has mixed reviews, with one study showing a correlation to increased CRP. I may have observed this in my own diet; when I was heavily using ghee in my diet, my CRP rose from 0.3mg/L to 0.8mg/L, still normal, but an increase. However, I generally felt fine eating large quantities of the stuff. Other studies show it is anti-inflammatory, body fat reducing, and cancer reducing.

Gamma linolenic acid (GLA) is an 18:3 (n-6) molecule that is considered anti-inflammatory, and produced in the body from LA. It can also be found in the diet in sources I would recommend like walnuts, flax, chia and hemp, but also in rapeseed, canola and soybeans. I've obtained copious amounts in my diet through flax (22.8 g/100 g) without noticing any negative effects. Walnuts are also very high in this good omega-6, but I would still recommend it in moderation, as it will interfere with absorption of the more valuable omega-3s.

Linoleic acid (LA) is an 18:2 (n-6) molecule that is essential. It is converted to GLA, and further converted to AA, and is therefore considered inflammatory. I believe it should be consumed minimally. It is present in high amounts in some foods that would otherwise be considered healthy, like hemp (25 g/100 g), walnuts (33 g/100 g), almonds (12 g/100 g), hazelnut (7.8 g/100 g), and others like poppy, sesame, safflower, sunflower, corn, soybean, peanut. Vegetable oils can have high content such as corn oil (53 g/100 g), soybean, safflower, sunflower (8.3 g/14 g, or 59 g/100 g), sesame, but also smaller quantities in healthier oils like olive (1.3 g/14 g or 9.3 g/100 g) and canola (2.6 g/14 g or 18.6 g/100 g). Nuts like sunflower, pine, pecan, brazil (9–6 g/serving), and cheeses like blue, brie (3–6 g/serving) all have significant amounts. Some healthy, low-starch grains also contain their fair share, like flax (5.9 g/100 g) and chia (5.8 g/100 g). Other meats and dairy are comparatively low, like chicken (2.9 g/100 g), Swiss cheese (0.6 g/100 g), milk (0.12 g/100 g) and beef (0.56 g/100 g). In my own personal experience, hemp and walnut in raw form seem to have no ill effect but seem to contribute to inflammation over a few days or week of consumption. If you're already consuming some healthy olive oil or flax in your diet, that should be plenty, and I would recommend avoiding further concentrated sources like many nuts, oils and nut butters.

Arachidonic acid (AA) is considered inflammatory. Its function is for muscle tissue inflammation. However, with regard to AS, I believe it should be avoided as much as possible. Prostaglandin E2 EP4 is a metabolite of AA, and directly contributes to the "bone remodelling and deposition" in AS. *"Individuals suffering from joint pains or active inflammatory disease may find that increased arachidonic acid consumption exacerbates symptoms, presumably because it is being more readily converted to inflammatory compounds. Likewise, high arachidonic acid consumption is not advised for individuals with a history of inflammatory disease, or who are in compromised health."* The study goes on to support the understanding that omega-3 completes for availability with omega-6 in the body, and excessive omega-6 may counter the anti-inflammatory effects of omega-3's. It also states that AA does not appear to have pro-inflammatory effects in healthy individuals. This is specifically an AS related concern. (Rhodes, 2015), (Li B1, 1994).

Personally, I did not experience any detrimental effect from the consumption of AA, or at least the effects were very mild and felt only after several days of the same high-AA content food. One of the higher sources, beef liver (AA content of 0.23 g/100

g) did not contribute to inflammation, but actually made me feel more energetic in the days to come because I believe its high iron content helped me with my anemia. Another high source is egg yolk (typically 0.14 g/100 g). Egg was always part of my diet (sometimes very much so, with five or six eggs a day), and I never saw any correlation between eggs and inflammation. Other foods with AA include chicken fat (0.08 g/100 g) duck fat, and beef sausages (0.045 g/100 g). Notice the quantities here. If I were to have one of my big, six-egg omelettes, I would be eating about 300 g of egg and ingesting 0.42 g of AA. In comparison, a handful of walnuts (half a cup) contains 13.2 g of LA, which the body can convert to AA. And if I'm getting a good solid serving of 2000 mg (2 g) of omega-6 by eating fish for lunch, the total amount of oil from the egg is only a quarter of what I ingested from the fish, and since omega-3s and omega-6s can compete with each other in the body, it looks like the walnuts might be the bigger problem. One handful just swamped the omega-3 intake from the fish by more than a factor of 6! This fit my observations with my own diet. While AA is the inflammatory omega-6 of bigger concern with AS, the quantities seem to be more important. Chicken, liver and egg never bothered me, but too many nuts were a big problem.

Another study to support this was one conducted to investigate the use of walnuts as an intervention for cancer. Mice were fed walnut oil as part of their diet, while a control group was fed the same proportion of corn oil in their diet. The mice had human breast cancer cells implanted, and the rate of growth was observed. The rate of growth in the mice fed the walnut oil was significantly slower. The study goes on to say that, *"the omega-3 content of the walnut diet was reflected in the significant decrease in arachidonic acid (omega-6 fatty acid) and significant increases in the omega-3 fatty acids, eicosapentaenoic and docosahexaenoic acids in the liver [101]."* (Hardman, Diet components can suppress inflammation and reduce cancer risk, 2014)

This is relevant, because the purpose of the study was to show that chronic inflammation is a contributor to cancer, much like AS. However, the focus was on walnut oil and the omega-3 content, which is certainly a factor, but it fails to mention the proportions of omega-6 oils. Corn oil, which fed to the control group of mice, contains nearly double the quantities of omega-6 LA (53 g/100 g vs. 33 g/100 g), and while walnuts do have high quantities of omega-3 ALA, they also have very high quantities of LA, which is competitive with other omega-3 oils in the diet. Furthermore, the corn oil contains negligible amounts of AA, yet it showed to contribute significantly more to inflammation, clearly indicating that dietary AA is not the factor at play here. A low-LA content is also important. While walnut oil is much healthier and less inflammatory than corn oil, there are still much better options with lower-LA content.

In my personal experience, even the effect from omega-6 was relatively small compared to starch, which was by far the bigger source of acute arthritis flare-ups. Omega-6 seemed to be a long-term, chronic contributor.

## Saturated fats

Saturated fats are fats that are "saturated" with hydrogen atoms; there are sufficient hydrogens bonded to carbon atoms that there are no or very few double carbon bonds left, unlike polyunsaturated or monounsaturated fats, whose properties are defined by the double bond they contain. This also makes saturated fats less reactive (less susceptible to rancidity) since they've already reacted with hydrogen and are already more stable.

Much attitude and understanding has changed regarding saturated fats. They are not the villains they were once made out to be. I discussed fat consumption with my GP, and she indicated that cholesterol and dietary cholesterol are only weakly associated. My cholesterol levels were testing normal. At one point, early after my diagnosis, I had one test where my liver enzymes were slightly elevated, and my GP recommended cutting back on fatty and spicy foods. It was also noted that elevated liver enzymes could be a side effect caused by liver damage from the medication. This was the only test I had that was out of range; once my medication was discontinued, for the following two years, my bi-monthly blood tests all returned normal, despite the increase of fats in my diet, including saturated fats from ghee. In my case at least, it seemed to show that the medication was more harmful in the long term than saturated fat (of course, in moderation).

As far as arthritis pain is concerned, saturated fats seemed to cause no contribution to AS. Probably the best saturated fat, coconut oil, may also help reduce arthritis as it is considered anti-inflammatory; sterols promote natural steroid hormones including corticosteroids which help control inflammation. This includes the popular MCT oil (medium-chain triglycerides), which are the medium-length chain fat molecules derived from coconut oil.

Below is a summary of lipids (fats) and their assessment in relation to arthritis. I've highlighted beneficial items in green, cautionary items in yellow, and items to avoid in red:

| Common name | Sources (both low and high examples) | Assessment |
|---|---|---|
| Conjugated Linoleic acid (CLA) | Ghee | Anti-inflammatory, body fat reducing, cancer reducing. This is an omega 6 but tends to act like an omega 3 in the body, however, one study shows a correlation to an increase in CRP. |
| Punic Acid - Isomer of (CLA) | Pomegranate | Anti-inflammatory, anti-prostate cancer, reduces perirenal and epididymal fat. Unregulates TNF expression, blocks COX enzyme activity which regulates production of prostaglandins. |
| Palmitoleic Acid (Omega 7) | macadamia nuts (13g/100g), Olive oil (1.2g/100g) | Healthy, anti-inflammatory. May promote insulin resistance, improved serum lipid profile. |
| Oleic Acid (Omega 9) | Olive oil (71g/100g), Avocado oil (67g/100g), Cocoa butter (32.5g/100g) macadamia nuts (43.7g/100g), avocado (9g/100g), Olives (7.7g/100g), olive oil, also high concentrations in pecan, canola, macadamia, and high oleic sunflower oil, Flax, swiss cheese (6g/100g), sprats (2.1g/100g), salmon (2g/100g) | Healthy, anti-inflammatory. May promote insulin resistance, improved serum lipid profile. "High levels of lipids in the bloodstream have the potential to ultimately reduce glucose uptake at any given level of insulin. This mechanism is quite fast-acting and may induce insulin resistance within days or even hours in response to a large lipid influx." In vivo, a high fat diet seems to have a lowering effect on insulin resistance. |
| Linoleic acid (LA) | -corn oil (53g/100g), hemp (25g/100g), walnut (33g/100g), almond (12g/100g) poppy, hazelnut (7.8g/100g), sesame, safflower, sunflower, corn, soybean, peanut.<br>-vegetable oils (sunflower (59g/100g), sesame, corn, olive (1.3g/14g, canola (2.6g/14g)<br>-nuts like sunflower, pine, pecan, brazil (9-6 grams/serving) Flax (5.9/100g), chia (5.8g/100g)<br>-Sprats (3.5g/100g)<br>-chicken (2.9g/100g), pork<br>-Salmon (.7g/100g)<br>-cheeses (0.6g/100g)<br>-Beef (.56g/100g) | Biosynthesis of Arachidonic acid (AA) and LA, however the correlation is dampened. In moderation ok, avoid excessive amounts. An essential fat, body converts to GLA which is good, but further converted to AA. **Inflammatory through AA.** Excessive amounts considered "not good for health", very high in peanuts. Suggested that 'various oxidized forms of LA" are directly responsible for stimulation inflammation. |
| α-Linolenic acid (ALA) | Chia, Flax, fish, hemp (10g/100g), walnut (2g/100g) | Converts to EPA. Anti-inflammatory, primarily for colon health. |

| Common name | Sources | Assessment |
|---|---|---|
| Linolenic (See ALA) | | |
| Gamma-linolenic acid (GLA) | Rapeseed canola, soybeans, walnuts, flax (22.8/100g), perilla, chia and hemp (2g/100g) | Produced from LA. Anti-inflammatory. |
| Arachidonic acid (AA, ARA) | - Duck egg (.31g/100g)<br>-Beef liver (.23g/100g)<br>-egg yolk (Born 3 has .14g/100g)<br>-Poultry (chicken, .08g/100g, duck, from the fat)<br>- Beef Sausages (.045g/100g)<br>-Red Meat (fat), lean ground beef has .039g/100g,<br>-Milk (0g/100g)<br>-cheeses ( 0g/100g)<br>-certain fish (tilapia has 0g/100g, sprats has 0g/100g catfish, yellowtail)<br>-corn oil, 0g | Muscle tissue inflammation. Avoid as much as possible. Inflammatory and anti-inflammatory. Prostaglandin E2 EP4 is a metabolite of AA, and directly contributes to the "bone remodelling and deposition" in AS. Indomethacin is a NSAID effective in AS for it's ability to inhibit prostaglandins, which may speak to the need to limit AA.<br><br>"Individuals suffering from joint pains or active inflammatory disease may find that increased arachidonic acid consumption exacerbates symptoms, presumably because it is being more readily converted to inflammatory compounds. Likewise, high arachidonic acid consumption is not advised for individuals with a history of inflammatory disease, or who are in compromised health. Of note, while ARA supplementation does not appear to have proinflammatory effects in healthy individuals, it may counter the anti-inflammatory effects of omega-3 fatty acid supplementation." |
| Eicosapentaenoic acid (EPA) | Fish, sprats (.7g/100g), salmon (.7g/100g) | Anti-Inflammatory. |
| Docosahexaenoic acid (DHA) | Fish, Salmon (1.4g/100g), sprats (.6g/100g) | Anti-Inflammatory. Obtain greater than 2g/day. |

| Common name | Sources | Assessment |
|---|---|---|
| Saturated Fatty Acids (SFA) | Various | The substitution of SFA with Mono-Unsaturated Fatty Acids or Poly Unsaturated Fatty Acids eliminates the proinflammatory activity of LPS. Macrophages, and other cells of the innate immune system, possess receptors that recognize LPS. LPS-mediated signaling through TLR4 leads to the activation of NF-κB, and turns on the expression of proinflammatory cytokines, such as TNF-α, IL-1, IL-6, and IL-8. Inflammation and Insulin Resistance following High Fat Diet are heavily influenced by dietary Saturated Fat content; however, these responses are not necessarily proportional to the SF percentage.** SFA's are ok in moderation, but keep quantities low to avoid inflammation. Avoid SFA's with long chains. |
| Butyric Acid | animal fat, plant oils, milk, butter parmesean cheese, and as a result of anaerobic fermentation. | Considered an SCT oil. Among the short-chain fatty acids, butyrate is the most potent promoter of intestinal regulatory T cells in vitro. It possesses both preventive and therapeutic potential to counteract inflammation-mediated ulcerative colitis and colorectal cancer. |
| Octanoic acid (Caprylic Acid) | Coconut (2.3g/100g), Butter (1g/100g) | Considered an MCT oil, can help in the process of excess calorie burning. |
| Decanoic acid (Capric Acid) | Cocount (10%) | Considered an MCT oil, can help in the process of excess calorie burning. |
| Dodecanoic acid (Lauric Acid) | Coconut (14.8g/100g), Butter (2.5g/100g), also found in breast milk | Considered an MCT oil, lauric acid has been characterized as having "a more favorable effect on total HDL cholesterol than any other fatty acid, either saturated or unsaturated". In some studies, results failed to demonstrate any significant impact of fat source on any biomarkers of inflammation. |
| Tetradecanoic acid (Myristic Acid) | Nutmeg butter (75%), Butter (7.4g/100g), Cocount (5.8g/100g), Cream (3.7g/100g), Swiss cheese (3g/100g), egg (.03g/100g) | As above, results in some studies failed to demonstrate any significant impact of fat source on any biomarkers of inflammation. |

| | | |
|---|---|---|
| **Hexadecanoic Acid (Palmitic acid)** | Palm oil (43g/100g), cocoa butter (25g/100g), butter/ghee (21.6g/100g), cream (9.7g/100g), swiss cheese (7.8g/100g), olive oil (11.2g/100g), avocado oil (11g/100g), macadamia nuts (6g/100g), coconut (2.8g/100g), egg (2.2g/100g), avocado (2g/100g), black olives (1.1g/100g), sprats (1g/100g) | According to the World Health Organization, evidence is "convincing" that consumption of palmitic acid increases the risk of developing cardiovascular disease, based on studies indicating that it may increase LDL levels in the blood. Increases in dietary PA (Palmitic) decrease fat oxidation and daily energy expenditure, whereas decreases in PA and increases in OA (Oleic) had the opposite effect. Increases in dietary PA may increase the risk of obesity and insulin resistance. Through raised adiposity levels, this could increase inflammation. |
| **Octadecanoic acid (Stearic acid)** | Animal fat, cocoa butter (33g/100g), shea butter, butter/ghee (10g/100g), cream (4.5g/100g), swiss cheese (3.2g/100g) coconut meat (1.7g/100g) | The fraction of dietary stearic acid that oxidatively desaturates to oleic acid is 2.4 times higher than the fraction of palmitic acid analogously converted to palmitoleic acid. Also, stearic acid is less likely to be incorporated into cholesterol esters. In epidemiologic and clinical studies, stearic acid was found to be associated with lowered LDL cholesterol in comparison with other saturated fatty acids. |

*References:*

*CLA reduces inflammation (Shane M Huebner, 2010). CLA increases CRP (HealthDay, 2017)CLA reduces body fat mass (Jean-Michel Gaullier, 2004). CLA role in prevention of cancer (Ki Won Lee, 2005). CLA inflammatory properties (M A Zulet, 2005). Oleic acid and insulin resistance (Clarke, 2020)ALA, flax seed (P W Wiesenfeld, 2003). ALA, fatty acids and inflammation (Fritsche, The Science of Fatty Acids and Inflammation, 2015). AA inflammation (Rhodes, Grapiprant: an EP4 prostaglandin receptor antagonist and novel therapy for inflammation, 2015). AA and omega 3's (B Li, 1994). Saturated fats and inflammation (Reilly T. Enos, 2013). Butyrate (Steven A. L. W. Vanhoutvin, 2009). Lauric acid and mysristic acid (Fritsche, The Science of Fatty Acids and Inflammation, 2015). Palmitic acid (C Lawrence Kien, 2005) (Gianfranca Carta, 2017)*

## Daily calories – food list

As I started to manage my diet more closely, I began to count not only calories, but carbohydrates, protein and fat intake as well. I eventually dropped that strategy; I wouldn't generally recommend counting calories. It can be overwhelming and time consuming, but I did learn much about how different foods compare in macro nutrients, and it helped with my strategy in developing a healthy, satisfying diet after eliminating starchy foods from my plate. Eventually, I adapted this list to focus on foods that had high nutrition density, low carbs, moderate protein and moderate fat.

Below is a list of some recommended foods based on their macronutrients (fat, protein and carbohydrates) and total calorie content. I've highlighted foods in green that I would recommend based on their anti-inflammatory properties, and that are also low energy density (low calorie per serving). Foods highlighted in yellow are also beneficial but should be eaten in moderation due to high calorie, carb or protein content.

Whole grains like flax, oats and high-fibre cereals are also digested less efficiently than we used to think. A recent study looked at what happened when volunteers consumed a whole-grain diet that included 30 g of dietary fibre versus a standard American diet that contained half as much fibre. An increased number of calories were lost to the feces, as well as a bump in metabolism. Most people get way too much, but sugars and carbs are not to be completely avoided. They help the body absorb many other nutrients, including tryptophan which the body uses to produce serotonin, which helps prevent depression.

| Food | Calories | Fat (g) | Protein (g) | Carb Intake (g) | Fibre | Insulin Effect | Serving size |
|---|---|---|---|---|---|---|---|
| apple | 116 | 0.4 | 0.6 | 31.0 | 5.0 | 26.3 | one, large |
| asparagus | 20 | 0.1 | 2.2 | 3.9 | 2.1 | 3.0 | 100g |
| avocado | 161 | 14.5 | 2.0 | 8.5 | 6.5 | 3.1 | 100g (half fruit) |
| bell pepper | 31 | 0.3 | 1.0 | 6.1 | 2.1 | 4.5 | 100g |
| blackberry | 43 | 0.5 | 1.4 | 10.0 | 5.0 | 5.8 | 100g |
| blueberry | 57 | 0.3 | 0.7 | 14.0 | 2.4 | 12.0 | 100g |
| bok choy | 13 | 0.2 | 1.5 | 2.2 | 1.0 | 2.0 | 100g |
| broccoli | 34 | 3.1 | 2.8 | 6.6 | 2.6 | 5.5 | 100g |
| brussels sprout | 43 | 0.3 | 3.4 | 9.0 | 3.8 | 7.0 | 100g |
| cabbage, red | 31 | 0.2 | 1.4 | 7.0 | 2.1 | 5.7 | 100g |
| cauliflower | 25 | 0.3 | 1.9 | 5.0 | 2.0 | 4.0 | 100g |
| celery | 16 | 0.2 | 0.7 | 3.4 | 1.6 | 2.2 | 100g |
| chard | 19 | 1.7 | 4.4 | 3.7 | 1.6 | 4.5 | 100g |
| cheese, swiss | 106 | 8.0 | 8.0 | 0.9 | 0.0 | 5.2 | 1 slice |
| chia | 170 | 10.0 | 7.0 | 13.5 | 11.0 | 6.3 | 32g |
| chicken broth | 36 | 1.2 | 2.5 | 3.9 | 0.0 | 5.2 | 100g |
| chicken meat | 239 | 14.0 | 27.0 | 0.0 | 0.0 | 14.6 | 100g |
| chocolate, dark | 170 | 14.0 | 4.0 | 7.7 | 4.0 | 5.9 | 85% cocao, 30g |
| coconut flour | 120 | 3.0 | 3.0 | 9.0 | 5.0 | 5.6 | 28g (1oz) |
| coconut water | 45 | 0.5 | 1.7 | 9.0 | 2.6 | 7.3 | 250ml |
| coconut wrap | 60 | 2.5 | 0.0 | 9.5 | 6.5 | 3.0 | 1 wrap |
| cod | 82 | 0.7 | 18.0 | 0.0 | 0.0 | 9.7 | 100g |
| cranberry, dried | 123 | 0.5 | 0.0 | 29.7 | 2.3 | 27.4 | 40g |
| cucumber / pickle | 15 | 0.1 | 1.6 | 3.6 | 0.5 | 4.0 | 100g |
| date ball, maca | 150 | 8.0 | 5.0 | 14.9 | 11.0 | 6.6 | per ball |
| egg | 78 | 5.0 | 6.0 | 2.5 | 0.0 | 5.7 | 1 large (50g) |
| figs | 43 | 0.3 | 1.3 | 8.8 | 2.0 | 7.5 | 100g |
| flaxseed | 134 | 10.5 | 4.5 | 5.8 | 7.0 | 1.2 | 25g |
| ghee | 112 | 12.7 | 0.0 | 0.0 | 0.0 | 0.0 | 1 tbsp |
| goji berries | 112 | 1.4 | 4.0 | 20.9 | 7.0 | 16.1 | 28g (1oz) |
| golden berries | 53 | 0.7 | 1.9 | 11.0 | 1.2 | 10.8 | 100g |
| grapes | 67 | 0.4 | 0.6 | 17.0 | 0.9 | 16.4 | 100g |

| | | | | | | | |
|---|---|---|---|---|---|---|---|
| green onion | 32 | 0.2 | 1.8 | 5.8 | 2.6 | 4.1 | 100g |
| halibut | 186 | 14.0 | 14.0 | 1.7 | 0.0 | 9.3 | 100g |
| hemp hearts | 170 | 13.0 | 10.0 | 3.9 | 1.2 | 8.1 | 30g |
| herring | 160 | 10.0 | 17.0 | 0.0 | 0.0 | 9.2 | 1 can (80g) |
| honey | 64 | 0.0 | 0.1 | 15.9 | 0.0 | 16.0 | 1 tbsp |
| kale | 50 | 0.7 | 3.3 | 10.0 | 2.0 | 9.8 | 100g |
| kefir (2% milk) | 124 | 4.9 | 8.0 | 12.2 | 0.0 | 16.5 | 1 cup (250ml) |
| kefir (homo milk) | 160 | 8.0 | 8.0 | 14.4 | 0.0 | 18.7 | 1 cup (250ml) |
| Kefir (water) | 3 | 0.0 | 0.0 | 0.8 | 0.0 | 0.8 | 250ml |
| kelp | 43 | | | 10.8 | 1.3 | 9.5 | 100g |
| kiwi | 61 | 0.5 | 1.1 | 14.7 | 3.0 | 12.3 | 100g (2 small fruit) |
| lettuce | 15 | 0.2 | 1.4 | 2.9 | 1.3 | 2.4 | 100g |
| liver, beef | 191 | 5.0 | 29.0 | 5.0 | 0.0 | 20.7 | 100g |
| macadamia nuts | 718 | 76.0 | 8.0 | 14.0 | 9.0 | 9.3 | 100g |
| mackerel in olive oil | 528 | 19.0 | 15.0 | 0.0 | 0.0 | 8.1 | 115g can |
| mayonnaise | 100 | 10.0 | 0.1 | 2.9 | 0.0 | 3.0 | 1tbsp |
| mushroom | 22 | 0.3 | 3.1 | 3.3 | 1.0 | 4.0 | 100g |
| mustard | 7 | 0.8 | 0.8 | 1.2 | 0.8 | 0.8 | 20g |
| oil, Coconut | 132 | 15.0 | 0.0 | 0.0 | 0.0 | 0.0 | 1 tbsp |
| oil, olive | 880 | 100.0 | 0.0 | 0.0 | 0.0 | 0.0 | 100g |
| oil, olive | 1100 | 125.0 | 0.0 | 0.0 | 0.0 | 0.0 | 125g |
| oil, olive | 132 | 15.0 | 0.0 | 0.0 | 0.0 | 0.0 | 1 tbsp |
| oil, omega 3 | 59 | 6.7 | 0.0 | 0.0 | 0.0 | 0.0 | 4 capsules |
| olives, black | 115 | 10.7 | 0.8 | 6.3 | 3.2 | 3.5 | 100g |
| onion | 40 | 0.1 | 1.1 | 9.0 | 1.7 | 7.9 | 100g |
| orange | 47 | 0.1 | 0.9 | 10.6 | 2.4 | 8.7 | 100g |
| pineapple | 50 | 0.1 | 0.5 | 13.0 | 1.4 | 11.9 | 100g |
| plum | 46 | 0.3 | 0.7 | 10.1 | 1.4 | 9.1 | 100g |
| pomegranate | 83 | 1.2 | 1.7 | 19.0 | 4.0 | 15.9 | 100g |
| prune | 240 | 0.4 | 2.2 | 64.0 | 7.0 | 58.2 | 100g |
| raisins | 129 | 0.2 | 1.3 | 34.0 | 1.6 | 33.1 | small box (43g) |
| raspberry | 53 | 0.7 | 1.2 | 12.0 | 7.0 | 5.6 | 100g |
| ricotta | 174 | 13.0 | 11.0 | 3.9 | 0.0 | 9.8 | 100g |

| | | | | | | | | |
|---|---|---|---|---|---|---|---|---|
| salmon, sockeye | 131 | 4.5 | 23.0 | 0.0 | 0.0 | 12.4 | 100g |
| sardines in olive oil | 391 | 37.6 | 15.6 | 0.0 | 0.0 | 8.4 | 106g can |
| shrimp | 99 | 0.3 | 24.0 | 0.0 | 0.0 | 13.0 | 100g |
| spinach | 23 | 0.4 | 2.9 | 3.6 | 2.2 | 3.0 | 100g |
| sprat | 208 | 11.0 | 25.0 | 0.0 | 0.0 | 13.5 | 100g |
| strawberry | 33 | 0.3 | 0.3 | 7.3 | 2.0 | 5.5 | 100g |
| tilapia | 129 | 2.7 | 26.0 | 0.0 | 0.0 | 14.0 | 100g |
| tomato | 18 | 0.2 | 0.9 | 3.9 | 1.2 | 3.2 | 100g |
| tomato sauce | 70 | 0.4 | 3.2 | 16.0 | 3.7 | 14.0 | 250ml |
| trout, canned, in olive oil | 430 | 42.0 | 15.0 | 0.0 | 0.0 | 8.1 | 106g can |
| tuna, albacore | 172 | 7.2 | 25.2 | 2.0 | 0.0 | 15.6 | 100g |
| whipping cream | 97 | 10.4 | 0.6 | 0.8 | 0.0 | 1.1 | 1oz (28g) |
| zucchini | 54 | 1.0 | 3.9 | 10.0 | 3.2 | 8.9 | 323g |

# CHAPTER 8

# DIET

*Dietary change is a key mechanism for reducing obesity and for providing components to suppress inflammation, decrease oxidative damage and change gene expression. It has been shown that at least part of the mechanism for suppression of carcinogenesis of many dietary components is by the suppressing the activation of NF-kB. (Hardman, Diet components can suppress inflammation and reduce cancer risk, 2014).*

Before the main onset of my arthritis, I had a very high-carb diet, which feeds the *Klebsiella* bacteria, I ate foods high in omega-6, which are inflammatory, and consumed emulsifiers in my diet from processed foods that have been linked to colon inflammation, so I was setup for high inflammation and gastrointestinal infection. From packaged cereals, pastas, pizza, peanut butter sandwiches, to finishing kids' cereals in evening, and a very early breakfast (5:00 a.m.), I was never hungry and always in a fed state. I suspect the final straw was my intestinal illness after my trip, which may have allowed *Klebsiella* to proliferate in my system.

After 18 months of trial and error with diets, including an elimination diet to reintroduce foods one at a time to test my body's reaction, here are a list of dietary recommendations I can make based on my own experience. I recommend you do your own elimination diet to determine which foods work best for you. In my recommended foods section, I include comments based on studies that indicate why or how some of these foods can be anti-inflammatory.

General Recommendations
- Very low-amylose starch (resistant starch that is normally not digested and is food for *Klebsiella*). Fructose and glucose are ok, but don't over-consume fruit. Limited simple carbs like sucrose, lactose, should be less than 5 g/serving). Amylopectin starch is ok in moderation (low-RS breads).
- Maintain diverse probiotic sources (kefir, sauerkraut, pickles in brine, blueberries, raspberries) to crowd out *Klebsiella*.
- Omega-3 fat from dietary or supplemental sources to reduce inflammation 3–5 g/day. (Patty W Siri-Tarino, 2010)
- Omega-3 ALA to protect from colon inflammation (flax oil, omega-3 eggs).
- Avoid omega-6 and trans fats due to their inflammatory nature.
- Ensure you get enough fibre (cellulose and lignin). Vegetables at every meal, especially kale and broccoli, green tea, garlic (allicin), rosemary (ursolic acid), other high-fibre foods (fibre is cellulose derived from plants and it is shown that *Klebsiella* does not grow on fibre, but instead derives sugars from the polysaccharide starch).
- No processed foods or ingredients, as they are generally inflammatory and you may find you have sensitivities to certain additives if you make a food diary.
- No alcohol; it's very inflammatory.

- 16:8 intermittent fasting—the hours I prefer are no food after dinner (8:00 p.m.) till breakfast at work (12:00 p.m.). This promotes cortisol and ketone body production.
- Gelatin/collagen for joint repair and healing.
- Maintain a relatively light digestive load! Eat a normal serving size, eat slowly, drink water with a meal to help avoid overeating. Wait for at least 30 minutes to see if I'm full. (I usually feel much fuller half-an-hour after a meal!) I feel that overeating may also result in undigested carbs, which can be food for *Klebsiella*, as overeating even safe foods has caused flare-ups.
- Meals with a balance of simple carbs (fruit and veggies), protein and fat seem to sit well, be satisfying and give balanced energy.
- Don't try to reduce fatigue by eating more. Drink water, get up and move around, or take a rest if needed.
- Keep dinner the smallest meal of the day. Avoid kefir in the evening to avoid bloating.
- Avoid grazing to avoid overeating and eat three reasonably portioned meals with breaks in between.
- Oils at wakeup are effective at staving off hunger and maintaining energy without breaking a fast or taking the body out of ketosis. Try MCT oil, oregano, olive, flax or fish oils.

Balanced Macros
- Moderate carbs to low carbs, and monosachharides (simple sugars) only. Avoid foods with resistant starch (RS) entirely.
- Protein, moderate quantities. Source from vegetables and fish. Try to limit animal and milk protein, as this is associated with Crohn's disease and Crohn's disease is associated with AS. Personally, low-lactose dairy products like Swiss cheese or kefir have been no problem for me,

but others I've spoken to with AS feel better staying away from dairy.
- Fat (remainder of calorie intake), mostly from fish (omega-3s (EPA, DHA)) including fish skin, coconut oil, and MCT oil. Allow saturated fats primarily from coconut. Monounsaturated fats from olive oil, avocados, macadamia nuts and whole milk kefir (some saturated from dairy is ok).

## Protein restriction

I have been often reminded by my relatives to feed my kids more meat. "Growing kids need protein!" is the phrase I usually hear. And it's ubiquitous in our current culture; protein bars, protein shakes, protein balls, on top of the high-protein foods we eat as a staple with every meal like fish, chicken shrimp or beef. But how much do we need? Many current sources state we need 0.7–0.8 g/kg of body weight. For myself, at 163 lbs, that means 59 g of protein. When tracking my protein (and other macros), I would regularly exceed this recommendation, often getting around 90 g of protein a day, but often 120 g, 130 g or even up to 175 g of protein in one day. This usually happened when I had a protein-rich food at each meal, like eggs for breakfast, fish at lunch and chicken at dinner. But even on more moderate days, when I ate a serving of fish and eggs at a later meal, I could easily be in the 120 g range. When I counted the protein from all my food, it really added up: 9 g from broccoli, 4.6 g from cauliflower, 8 g from a slice of Swiss cheese, 7 g from chia, and 10.5 g from almonds. Much of what I was eating on its own was a complete or near complete protein from vegetarian sources. It was often believed that too much was not a problem, but more recent studies show that it can have negative effects for general health:

> *Low protein intake is associated with a major reduction in IGF-1, cancer, and overall mortality*

> *in the 65 and younger but not older population. These results suggest that low protein intake during middle age followed by moderate to high protein consumption in old adults may optimize health span and longevity (Levine ME1, 2014) and for weight loss (Cyrus Khambatta, 2018).*

Protein has an influence on metabolism and on blood glucose levels. In relation to AS, it may also have an impact. Once study showed that high-protein diets increase oxidative stress:

> *"In addition, the normal-protein group experienced a reduction in oxidative-stress-related metabolic processes after losing weight, but the high-protein group did not see this improvement. The normal-protein group also saw decreased gene expression of genes associated with oxidative stress, while the high-protein group increased the expression of genes associated with oxidative stress. The authors hypothesized that this increase in oxidative stress may explain why the high-protein diet negated the improvements in insulin sensitivity typically observed with weight loss." (MJ1., 1997).*

As mentioned before, oxidative stress has been identified as a contributor to arthritis and cancer, so it may be beneficial to keep your protein intake moderate.

## Calorie restriction and total energy expenditure

Energy in must equal energy out. The conservation of energy in an isolated system is the first law of thermodynamics. It makes sense in physics, engineering, and chemistry, so why shouldn't it also apply to biology? It has always been assumed that if the total amount of energy gained in the body through food equals the amount burned (or expended) through base metabolic processes plus calories burned through physical activity, a person's weight will be stable. Add 200 calories to the diet from broccoli and burn 200 calories more on the treadmill. Add 800 calories to the diet from donuts and burn 800 more calories on the treadmill. Right? Makes sense intuitively, but modern research is proving this concept to be wrong.

It turns out that the body's total energy expenditure (TEE) does not increase linearly in this fashion. Many studies are now showing that physical activity can be increased, and the body's TEE increases correspondingly at first, but then levels off. At high levels of physical activity, the body's TEE is lower than what has been traditionally expected; it doesn't increase as much as the increase in physical activity, but the treadmill isn't lying. It turns out that running four hours on the treadmill does take more energy than running for two hours. The body can't increase TEE indefinitely, so it reduces the base metabolic rate (the calories your body uses when at rest) instead to obtain the required energy to complete the run. This has impact on normal body functions, including a reduction in somatic (tissue) repair, and a reduction in reproductive system activity. Too much is a bad thing, especially when it comes to tissue repair, but there is evidence that the right balance of activity may temper an overactive immune system.

> *"Although metabolic responses to increased PA may frustrate exercise-based weight loss programs, the reduction in non-PA metabolic activity in response to increased PA appears to be a critical mechanism by which exercise protects against chronic disease (23,25). In a Constrained TEE model, increased exercise is expected to reduce non-PA metabolic activity, which may in turn reduce inflammatory or endocrine response*

> *to pathogens and other physical or psychological stressors. Indeed, the anti-inflammatory benefits of exercise are well documented (25), and exercise has been shown to reduce inflammation related to cardiovascular disease risk (e.g., C-reactive protein; 17) and rheumatic disease (2)." (Pontzer, 2015)*

Other studies confirm these findings. Not only does exercise build strength and burn fat, but it reduces the amount of caloric energy available for other inflammatory processes, having a direct impact on autoimmune diseases. (U.S. Department of Health & Human Services, 2009)

However, be patient! Calorie restriction, as a therapeutic treatment to reduce inflammation, requires commitment over a longer period of time, likely a year or a couple years. It should be viewed as a change in lifestyle for best reductions in CRP and TNFα reductions. In the study, inflammatory markers showed a persistent reduction, with no corresponding reduction in immune response, which is a common side effect of many medications prescribed for arthritis. Reductions in weight, fat mass and leptin were most pronounced after 12 months. (Gallagher S., 2016) Now those are side effects that I'd be happy to have.

Exercise is certainly beneficial if you have arthritis. Stretching, keeping the joints limber with a full range of motion, and building muscle strength to support the joints are more obvious aspects. But it turns out exercise, in conjunction with appropriate calorie restriction or fasting, seems to keep metabolic processes like inflammation under control as well. In my experience, it seems most appropriate to establish a healthy, moderate activity level with low-impact activities appropriate for your type of arthritis. This sets the physical activity energy expenditure. Then your calorie consumption, including diet and fasting, can be adjusted to provide good nutrition, but a slightly calorie-restricted diet, to help keep metabolic processes balanced and under control.

## Specific carbohydrate diet, fermentation and FODMAP

Earlier in my dietary testing and investigation, I came across the SCD and gave it a try. The SCD is based on the idea of limiting the diet to foods that require minimal digestive processes and leave virtually no material in the intestine. This seemed to be a great fit to be applied to AS, in the effort to limit starches in the gut that can feed *Klebsiella*. It focuses on simple sugars that are quickly digested. For example, fruit, containing monosaccharides glucose and fructose would be acceptable. Table sugar, sucrose, is a disaccharide and would be easily digestible.

This diet I found was very close to an ideal diet for AS, however, there were still foods that did not fit the correct pattern. For example, cashew was on the safe foods list in this diet, but I found that they repetitively contributed to increased arthritis pain. I suspected that the starch content in cashew was too high. Cocoa powder was on the "illegal" list of not-acceptable foods, but I was able to consume this with no problems. Cream is on the illegal list, but these were also fine for me in moderate amounts. Flax seed, also on the illegal list, also caused no problems.

One of the biggest differences I noticed were the cautions about inulin fibre. In the SCD, inulin is on the illegal foods list, and specifically mentioned as a potential food for *Klebsiella* in the gut. Before reading this, I added inulin to my diet, usually just when fasting, to avoid constipation. I've added it at other times to my diet as well, with no noticeable negative effects relating to arthritis pain, but I have noticed if I take too much, it does make the bowels move too fast and can contribute to flatulence or diarrhea. In general, I don't believe inulin is required if you are following a healthy, natural diet containing plenty of vegetables, and supplying natural fibre.

Also similar is the FODMAP diet, which stands for fermentable oligosaccharides, disaccharides, monosaccharides and polyols, which is the list of a group of carbohydrates that are known for triggering digestive symptoms like bloating, gas and stomach pain. A diet low in fermentable carbs, known as FODMAPs, is clinically recommended for the management of irritable bowel syndrome (IBS). FODMAPs are found in a wide range of foods in varying amounts. Some foods contain just one type, while others contain several. The main dietary sources of the four groups of FODMAPs include:

- Oligosaccharides: Wheat, rye, legumes and various fruits and vegetables, such as garlic and onions.
- Disaccharides: Milk, yogurt and soft cheese. Lactose is the main carb.
- Monosaccharides: Various fruits including figs and mangoes, and sweeteners such as honey and agave nectar. Fructose is the main carb.
- Polyols: Certain fruits and vegetables including blackberries and lychee, as well as some low-calorie sweeteners like those in sugar-free gum.

This diet is not very different than the SCD, and I discovered it shortly after, but abandoned it very quickly as an option because it included starch as one of the safe foods. There were also other grains and flours that I knew caused a problem for me, including rice and other foods that were listed as safe on these diets but were generally inflammatory and resulted in increased inflammation, like peanut butter. High FODMAP foods that have given me no trouble include asparagus, avocado, broccoli, cauliflower, celery, seaweed, and zucchini. The cruciferous vegetables in particular I have long eaten in large quantities with no ill effects. Otherwise, the FODMAP diet contains many common foods with the low-starch, low-inflammation diet that worked for me in controlling AS and these two diets were very close to what I would recommend for AS. It may work for you if you have a different type of arthritis but still suffer from IBS symptoms.

## Gluten-free and lectin-free diet

A gluten-free diet involves excluding all foods from the diet that include gluten. Predominately this includes wheat, but also other grains like rye and barley. When investigating this diet as a solution to arthritis, I also found it close to what would work to help reduce AS symptoms, but there were some important differences. Most importantly, I saw that I was able to reintroduce refined white flour with amylase enzymes, which is something I would not be able to do if I had a gluten intolerance or sensitivity. But, at least superficially, a gluten-free diet and a diet appropriate for managing AS symptoms are really not that different. Grains like most wheat-based foods, rye and barley are commonly excluded. However, for those that are gluten intolerant, quinoa, rice, corn, potatoes and tapioca can be included in the diet, but for the AS suffer, these can all be problematic foods. The reason for the difference, again, is starch.

The lectin-free diet (gluten is a type of lectin) didn't fit my observations for AS either. In some similar diets, seeds like chia and vegetables like tomato and zucchini were not recommended (I had no issues with them). Macadamia nuts are recommended, but so are pistachios, while I found pistachios were only tolerable in small amounts, fitting an amylose starch theory more closely. Refined starches like white flour with amylase or glutenous rice, caused me no problems. Again, I'm not recommending the rice and flour as they have a high glycemic index and are not the healthiest of foods, but they certainly caused no problems with AS flare-ups. However, in interviewing a patient with Hashimoto's disease, this diet was very beneficial for her, so take this into account for your own situation.

## Low-starch diet

In 1996, both Dr. A. Ebringer and C. Wilson completed a paper entitled "The use of a Low Starch Diet in the Treatment of Patients Suffering from Ankylosing Spondylitis." It detailed the links between the HLA-B27 gene, and the elevated levels of total serum IgA, suggesting a bacterial microbe was acting across the gut mucosa in the intestine. Due to the similarity between HLA-B27 and *Klebsiella*, *Klebsiella* was the leading suspect. It went on further to state that by reducing food availability to the bacteria in the gut by resorting to a low-starch diet, IgA was reduced, as well as inflammation and symptoms in AS patients, and that further investigation was required into a low-starch diet.

This is what I intended to do, using my own condition as a test platform. The low-starch diet, as far as content is concerned, was by far the most effective diet in controlling AS symptoms. As mentioned before, amylose starch has shown itself as the number one contributor to arthritis pain and inflammation. The effect from amylose starch is clearly distinct from amylopectin, or other dietary fibres like inulin and cellulose. While I go on to recommend adding anti-inflammatory foods and other foods that reduce gut inflammation in general, the low-starch diet is probably the single most effective change you can make to your diet as an AS sufferer.

## Ketogenic diet

The ketogenic diet is another diet that makes for a very good general fit for arthritis sufferers. Originally, this diet was developed as a therapy for epilepsy. I originally tried it for the reported anti-inflammatory benefits, as discussed in chapter 4. Also, being a very low-carb diet, it serendipitously provided me benefit as an AS sufferer because it was naturally a low-starch diet. It most certainly helped me in my recovery from AS symptoms by helping me avoid starch, broke my fear of adding (healthy) fat to my diet, and helped establish healthy, moderate levels of protein intake. However, my diet eventually began to zero in on starch. While the ketogenic diet offered therapeutic benefit by suppressing macrophage activity, there were beneficial "non-keto" foods that was omitting from my diet, such as apple (apple skins contain allicin) and highly antioxidant foods like pomegranate, goldenberries or blueberries. A ketogenic diet was great for a while, but I felt that I often wanted to reintroduce foods like certain healthy fruits. The most beneficial fruits are also relatively low in sugar, so a moderately ketogenic diet is not necessarily incompatible with some fruit (mostly berry) consumption. While I would not consider myself to currently be on a ketogenic meal plan, I was on one for a good portion of my recovery, and it was certainly beneficial in the same way fasting was, and I would certainly use it again if my symptoms were to worsen. But now that my symptoms are relatively under control, I have been using fasting as a dietary maintenance tool and allowing myself some healthy fruits or grains like chia in my diet.

## 20:4 fasting, OMAD diet

A single, meal-a-day type of diet isn't a new idea. Ori Hofmekler was an early proponent for this diet. He was a member of the Israeli Defense Forces. The diet, simply put, allows for minimal eating during the day, and limiting eating to one main meal when one has more opportunity to rest, typically at the end of the day. He describes how the idea came to him:

> "I found out that some of my friends and I were doing much better when we reduced the eating during the day, or active time, and ate during the time when we knew that we could rest. I realized that when I ate the traditional 6 to 7 army meals plus snacks, I got more exhausted than ever. I suffered from energy crashes and my brain was not as focused and alert as I wanted it to be. . . . I felt a tremendous difference when I reduced drastically the amount of food I consumed during the day. Later when I went on to university and started my career as an artist, I realized that when I minimize eating during the day and have one main meal, I feel much more creative; much more alert. . . . After doing some research, I found out that other warriors of the past used to live like this and that is where I really got intrigued."

There are many variations now on the same theme, including 20:4 fasting (eating only within a four-hour window each day) or OMAD (one meal a day, eating once within a one-hour window). Most diets are focused on weight loss but of course in the context of this book we are trying to reduce symptoms associated with arthritis. This diet seemed to me to be the next best step after 16:8 fasting, just extending the fasting a little further each day.

At first it was a bit difficult, not because of the duration of the fasting period, but because I'm a "feaster," so once I start eating I like to keep eating, I like the sensation of being full. My problem initially was overeating, feeling like I needed to compensate, and giving myself permission to eat a day's worth of food in one meal. Of course, this led to a very full feeling, and bloating, which made my symptoms worse on many occasions. It took a few tries, but once I got this overeating under control, I was quite comfortable with a 20- or 22-hour fasting period each day. I would most often follow this routine during the week, when I could take advantage of not having to worry about breakfast or lunch during a busy day of work. I would relax my schedule on the weekends and enjoy a few extra meals with my family, usually shifting back to a 16:8 schedule. With this routine, I was never short on calories. The 20:4 during the week felt therapeutic for my arthritis and equality therapeutic for my gut—once I got used to the routine, I felt like I was never ready or wanting to eat before mid-afternoon anyway. I noticed some fleeting hunger pangs in the morning and a nice, clearing, cleansing sort of hunger pang in the afternoon, with the sensation that my gut was now ready to accept food again.

I feel like an eating schedule like this, with sufficient fasting time between periods of eating, was instrumental in giving my gut a chance to recover from the efforts of digestion from the day before.

*"It's when you eat that makes what you eat matter."*
—Ori Hofmekler

With a focus on micronutrients (vitamins and minerals through vegetables first, and a secondary focus on macronutrient balance, like protein, fat and carbs) I was making sure my weekday evening meals were heavy on fresh, raw or lightly steamed vegetables, healthy anti-inflammatory oils, and moderate levels of protein, which often included sources like fish, cheese and kefir and dips made with freshly ground flax. It took me a while to get used to this routine of eating, but it was a nice regimen, especially for weekdays, and felt beneficial for AS and for the gut. But if you have my eating habits, just watch out for evening bingeing.

## Alternate-day fasting

Another alternative could be alternate-day fasting (ADF). On fasting days, limit your dietary intake to less than 25% your caloric requirements; 500 calories for women and 600 calories for men. Alternate this with regular eating days so you don't feel limited to what you can eat, but do stick to a healthy diet. While this sounds more difficult at first, I actually found this relatively easy, as any cravings could simply be put off until tomorrow. Under this style of eating, I felt I developed a healthier relationship with food, and I had less temptation to binge on feeding days.

# CHAPTER 9

# MIND AND MUSCLE

**Exercise**

If you suffer from arthritis, a daily exercise routine is a must. Make it a habit. Once established, habits are easier to stick to on those mornings when you have trouble motivating yourself. Wake up in the morning and stretch, do Pilates, ride your bike, swim, or whatever works for you. I've found daily movement so important to maintaining range of motion, especially those days you don't feel like doing anything. I'm an avid cyclist, riding to and from work every day, and many days I didn't feel like riding, but I never regret it and always feel the benefit once I complete my ride. Every ride became a small victory in the battle over my AS. As I became stronger, some days I remember almost crying with joy at the end of my ride, happy that I was physically able to push myself like this again and be making progress. On these days when I arrived home, I would tell my wife that I had a million-dollar bike ride, it felt that good. A million dollars couldn't buy you that euphoria and pain relief. That joy, I'm sure, contributed to my health as well.

Becoming more active needs to fill your entire day. This was difficult for me, because I have a sedentary desk job, and a long commute, spending close to two hours in the car each day. Now I ride my bike to work (usually half the distance by car, then the rest by bike, due to the distance), I do weights and stretches, sit on a Swiss ball at work, use a standing desk (that can be raised and lowered so I can still spend some time on the Swiss ball), intentionally take the stairs whenever I can, and walk whenever I can.

If you have a sedentary job like I do, and your employer is willing to accommodate a little, a standing desk is a great option. There are many that are on the market these days, and one that can be raised and lowered is a great advantage, because as you probably know with AS, keeping the same position for too long is painful. Being able to stand for a while is beneficial, but being able to alternate throughout the day between sitting is better. I very rarely stand still; shifting my weight back and forth, even marching on the spot for a while helps. It might look funny, but constantly moving feels good for the back, feet and neck. At home, on my feet cooking or cleaning the kitchen, I'm doing the same thing, often to music. Dancing, twisting the back, raising the arms, turning the neck, plus a little rhythm from the music, is another great low-impact way to keep the back flexing.

Having said that, moderation is just as important. Natural body weight exercises are great at avoiding over-straining your joints. Exercise bands are also great at avoiding injury, only providing as much resistance and you can supply. Increasing weights to build muscle is generally a good idea since the muscle will go a long way in supporting the joints. In my teenage years, I would be sore the day after a workout with weights. This would be my recovery day, and I would feel great the day after. Now, the soreness after this type of resistance can typically last three days, and if I'm not careful, can cause a flare-up in my back, neck or shoulders.

Exercise is inflammatory and is the body's natural way of repair, but for us with arthritis, too much turns into another flare-up.

I have a short list of my favourite activities for AS—activities that I've felt have really benefited my condition over the years and continue to provide a therapeutic effect better than the best medication. Above all, avoid trauma, heavy impact, or repetitive strain. An injury in my twenties, plus stubbing my toe on my left foot in 2016, was evidence of arthritis induced by trauma. I felt on several occasions that I had very slow-healing injuries that would swell significantly and stay swollen for a long period of time, probably due to overactive inflammation in the body.

My most recommended activities are full body movement, in this order:

## *Swimming*

I always feel fantastic after a good swim. After a couple consecutive days of swimming, I forget for a while that I ever heard of anything called AS. It is a wonderful reprieve when you wake up in pain every morning. Swimming while camping for a week was very therapeutic; if I could only find the time in the day to swim every morning. I do my best to substitute, even "simulated swimming motions" on a Swiss ball for my morning stretches works well. Another option is on the treadmill, using some relatively light weights, swinging my arms and twisting my back rhythmically in swimming motion feels just as good. In my more severe stages of the condition, swimming was also a great activity for range of motion and a low-impact workout, alternating with lanes at the pool and the heat of the hot tub worked great on loosening joints and helping extend range of motion.

### Rowing

The upper body and shoulder exercise, gentle impact, and variable resistance feels great for my shoulders, back and chest range of motion. Also, there is some moderate benefit for the neck.

### Pilates

My general practitioner taught me that the muscles, when strengthened, can make up for and support weak or injured joints. In the very early stages of the onset of my AS, I underwent physiotherapy, with exercises mostly focusing on core strengthening, and in introduction to the Swiss ball. It served as a good introduction to Pilates. Pilates is a focus on core strengthening, including abdominal muscles and back muscles. I also included in my daily routine abdominal exercises, deep breathing, lots of daily stretching and range of motion exercises. It provided good gradual benefit and an exercise that I could fit in most any time and any place. I even can fit in a few exercises on the Swiss ball at work during my lunch break.

### Stretching

AS has affected my neck just as much as my mid-back and lumbar. The stiffness in this area was not present during the initial onset of AS but grew slowly and insidiously after I discontinued the use of sulfasalazine. Stretching and correcting my posture helped keep neck stiffness and pain at bay, especially when sitting at work and in the car. Keeping my head back and my chin in, proper upright posture sitting on the Swiss ball, and stretching my neck and back side to side, back and front, and arching my back forward and backward 8, 10 or 12 times a day continues to be beneficial. The more I move, the better I feel. It can be hard to start moving at times, but once I get going, I feel better and never regret the effort.

I've put so much effort into my daily stretching that I'm now more flexible than I was when I was doing track in high school. The increased range of mobility keeps the joints limber and reduces the chance of injury.

### Resistance exercises

Weights, push-ups, free-body shoulder and back exercises every day were and still are a big benefit. The weights were a good transition from Pilates, which focus on weightless exercises. Starting with 5 lb weights and slowly working up to 35 lbs, in combination with stretching, helped me push the joints and tendons slowly and gradually while at the same time rebuilding muscle strength. Squats and lunges help to work glutes and strengthen SI joint area of the lower back, including deadlifts. Daily push-ups gradually helped improve my mid- and upper-back.

### Cycling

This is a great, low-impact exercise and I've always been an avid cyclist. But I eventually had to admit that it wasn't the best activity for AS. On longer duration rides, by back would get sore sitting in the arched position. Also, I could not heal my plantar fasciitis for the longest time, until I took a four-week break from cycling. What I thought was arthritis in the foot behaved more like an overuse injury. I eventually started noticing that it improved with rest, while my back improved with exercise and became worse with rest, a clear hallmark sign of arthritis. Once I started to treat the plantar fasciitis as an injury, separate from the arthritis, it recovered. This included foot stretches (toes up, scrunches), shoe inserts and soft, roomy shoes with a large toe box and low heel, and most importantly, rest.

It's important to stay very active, but beware overuse injuries, as the inflammation associated with AS can just make a typical injury worse. A low-impact but very active lifestyle is a must; one that will keep you moving throughout the day, every day. Incorporate some rest days. Waking up early and doing stretches and getting on the bike to get moving was often the best way to start the day. However, once I started feeling good enough to sleep through the night without waking up in pain, rest days on the weekends were great and felt like they gave my joints a little extra time to heal from the increasing intensity I was adding to my workouts.

## Mind and spirit

I've found maintaining a positive attitude very important in my battle with AS. There are a couple reads that I can recommend in this area. The first is *You are the Placebo, Making your mind Matter*, by Dr. Joe Dispenza. From this book I'm reminded that attitude is everything, and it gave me the belief that yes, I can conquer AS. The book made a few specific references to AS cases, which hit me close to home and motivated me even more to focus on my own recovery. The placebo effect has always been of interest to me. It can attest to the great power of our minds to help us get well. Studies conducted on medications are always compared to placebos, but rarely do you get to hear how effective the placebo can be. In a study of sulfasalazine used for treating psoriatic arthritis, the patient's assessment of joint improvement was "clearly better" for 50% of patients taking the drug. How well did the placebo work? Thirty-seven percent of patients felt "clearly better," even though they were taking a placebo. (B Combe 1, 1996) This is the power of the mind. Just to make you think more about this effect, for the patients receiving the actual sulfasalazine, how many of them felt better just because they knew they were taking a pill? The difference between the placebo and sulfasalazine group is only 13%, if that's any indication.

Another recommendation is *When the Body Says No*, by Gabor Mate, M.D. This one was full of examples on how negative stress in your life can have a very strong correlation with health issues, again including examples specific to arthritis and AS. It was a good reminder to learn how to manage the stress in my life and prevent its contribution to AS. Dr. Mate also made mention to a "Non-complaining Stoicism" often exhibited by rheumatoid patients, which he felt was a contributing factor, and which I could definitely relate to in my own situation. Fortunately for me, in hindsight, I feel that my ability to push through things without complaint was also what helped me stick to new diets and daily exercise that helped me recover.

Coincidentally (or perhaps providentially), shortly after writing this about myself, I read the article called "Emotional Factors and Rheumatoid Arthritis" which I thought explained my situation quite well,

> *"The onset of arthritis in many instances was associated with loss of support, such as" (a) death of husband or wife; (b) separation from husband or wife; (c) prolonged separation from family; (d) leaving home to become established. It will be noted that these situations could produce acute and short periods of emotional stress on the one hand, or chronic prolonged stress on the other. Regarding the individual personalities it is rather difficult to generalize. However, many of these patients tended to be immature and dependent; they usually tried overly hard to please both in professional and social contacts, and either concealed hostility or expressed it indirectly. Many of them were rather perfectionistic and ambitious. This trait is actually an asset in the treatment program, if controlled, as they are often*

> *more zealous and productive in a rehabilitation program than might be expected, considering their physical disability." (Robinson, 1957).*

I won't go into to too many specifics, but much of this described me to a tee. I was fortunate to have the opportunity to be involved in a video with Arthritis Research Canada to help promote awareness of the link between anxiety, depression and arthritis and it can be found on their website at https://www.arthritisresearch.ca/arthritis-research-education-series/anxiety-depression/videos/.

My strategy, related to mind, spirit and emotion, included the following:

- A focus on optimism. Take things one day at a time, at the same time remember that these individual, daily battles will add up and bring you closer to health. In a time period of six months, it's amazing what new habits we can develop and become acclimatized to, including the appreciation for new healthy foods and flavours, new exercises and activities.
- Stress management, relaxation breathing, meditation, or time with the dog in a quiet environment or hiking on the trail.
- Daily humour. I can sometimes be humourless, and reminding myself to smile, laugh, and appreciate all the good in my life was a big help in changing my attitude. Laughter is medicine.
- Establishing some life goals and a strategy to bring them about (including sharing my experience in a book!).
- Connecting with others. Sharing your experiences and challenges, both for support, and to support others.

Here are some other interesting additional quotes relating to a patient's mindset when dealing with an illness:

> "What do you think might lie at the root of your illness? What does your body need in order to heal?... But more often than not, they said introspective things, like 'I hate my job,', 'I need more 'me' time,', 'I have to finish my novel, I need to hire a nanny, I need to make more friends, I need to forgive myself, I need to love myself, I need to stop being such a pessimist'." (Rankin, 2013)

> "... My bravest patients made radical changes. Some quit their jobs. Others left their marriages. Some moved to new cities or towns. Others pursued long-suppressed dreams. The results these patients achieved were astonishing. Sometimes, a list of illnesses would disappear, often quickly. Even smaller steps, like talking to a boss about workplace problems or seeing a marriage counselor helped. I was in awe." (Rankin, 2013)

## Circadian clock

There is a very clear and well-known time cycle to AS pain and stiffness. Pain typically increases in the evening, is felt overnight and at wakeup, and subsides in the morning. Earlier, when the disease activity was more severe, it would take all morning for the pain to ease. When disease activity was less, it would clear within an hour. Once symptoms were managed and I was off medication, usually after noon I would suffer no pain at all. I would always note that I felt my best in the day after my afternoon bike ride, around 4:00 p.m.

I also noticed subtleties when the pain was worst in the morning. Some weekend mornings, when I allowed myself to sleep in (past sunrise, 7:00 a.m.) I could, on occasion, almost sleep through the morning pain. Early weekday mornings when I was up at 5:00 a.m., pain would be scale one, then 6:00 am, once I was at work, it would be slightly worse at scale one to two. This would occur whether I drove to work or biked to work, so it seemed independent of my activity. It would then clear up gradually over the course of the morning, mostly within the first hour. This clearing time was also required on the weekends if I was up early and active on my feet or sitting on my chair at work. My activity or diet would change the intensity of pain, but the time-dependent daily cycle remained present. The cycle time seemed to correlate more closely to the time of day then the time of my sleep, since the pattern of pain did not follow changes to my sleep pattern. Waking naturally at sunrise feels best. When I was camping (when exposed directly to the natural light of the day), falling asleep at sunset and rising and sunrise felt very good the whole trip. I noticed a trend that if I woke up gradually, as natural daylight increased (either by sleeping outside during camping or leaving the blinds open in the bedroom) that I could bypass or sleep through some of the morning stiffness.

Other times, when I had a large dinner especially with suspect foods, I would feel worse in the evening after dinner than overnight or the next morning. There is a correlation to mealtime that was occurring as a secondary cycle overtop the correlation to time of day.

Other daily trend I noticed was feeling better after staying up a little late, which may explain a reduced melatonin production on a particular night. Light sleep often contributed less to stiffness, while a heavier sleep contributed more. At first, I assumed this was due to lack of movement (less tossing and turning) while sleeping, but the amount of melatonin secretion may also be a factor here. I was on several occasions able to correlate a "heavier" sleep with more morning stiffness.

What is causing all of this? It seems that melatonin is the factor. One study, shows that *"Ankylosing Spondylitis patients have higher melatonin levels and the melatonin levels of AS patients are associated with the duration of morning stiffness, disease activity, quality of life and enthesitis scores."* (S. Hizmetli1, 2015)

"Serum MLT (melatonin) levels were significantly increased in AS patients as compared to healthy controls …Thus, it seems that MLT levels reflect the disease activity in AS patients." (Senna MK1, 2012) But is melatonin inflammatory? It seems to increase disease activity by acting through cytokine production. Melatonin has been found to increase the production of IL-1, IL-6, TNFα and ROS (reactive oxygen species). As mentioned earlier, TNFα is considered a strong contributor to AS activity, and is a primary focus in pharmacy, with most AS drugs designed to act as TNFα antagonists. Even NSAIDS like naproxen suppress melatonin levels at night and in this way may contribute to lessened symptoms. In the earlier discussion about cytokines, it was noted that a beneficial increase in IL-10 will suppress inflammatory aspects of IL-1, IL-6 and TNFα, while we now see that melatonin seems to be doing the opposite. (V Srinivasan, 2005), (Carrillo-Vico A1, 2006)

Melatonin is a potent antioxidant that is produced naturally by humans in the pineal gland and it is also produced by plants. In humans, melatonin has a wide variety of endocrine, neural and immune functions. Melatonin has been shown to be protective against prostate, pancreatic, breast and colon cancer by multiple mechanisms, including reducing oxidative stress and inflammation, allowing the body to kill off sick or old cells (apoptosis) and inhibit the creation of new blood vessels (angiogenesis) which needs to be moderated in the body. (Hardman, Diet components can suppress inflammation and reduce cancer risk, 2014)

So, what can we do to manage our circadian rhythm and exposure to melatonin to manage our arthritis? Increase blue light before bed to reduce the melatonin that may be prepping our body for a night of pain and stiffness? I can't recommend this, because of all the other health detriments associated with losing good quality sleep. But I did notice that red light, while it did not have such a pronounced effect on melatonin, is reported to increase cortisol production overnight, which could be used beneficially for AS symptoms without other side effects, much like staying up late around the campfire while camping, or like our ancient ancestors may have done. Once I was able to sleep well enough through the night and had a good exercise and stretching routine during the day, a longer sleep felt just fine, usually beneficial when I was able to wake up naturally with the daylight. Sufficient sleep is certainly a key factor in any kind of recovery.

Other factors to consider when trying to manage your melatonin levels:

- Foods: Melatonin is highest in rice and barley. It is also high in olive oil, but the oleocanthal still seems to provide net benefit.
- Fasting: "Strong influence of food on melatonin synthesis is detected in studies of subjects undergoing periods of fasting. Energy restriction reduces the nocturnal secretion of melatonin although the number of human studies proving this is limited." and "Melatonin secretion is strongly related to the duration of darkness."(Katri Peuhkuri, 2012)

# CHAPTER 10

# GENERAL MANAGEMENT AND SOLUTIONS

## What worked? What didn't? (Assessment of treatment effectiveness)

Over the course of a full year, I tabulated data from my daily log, and categorized some of the main factors that I changed in my lifestyle. They include the exclusion of amylose starch and refined starches (mostly white flour) in my diet, the use of a strict diet including intermittent and extended fasting as a therapeutic tool to manage flare-ups, the use of inflammatory foods, and the use of both intense and light/moderate exercise activity.

Using a statistical analysis commonly used in engineering called a Design-Of-Experiments, I used the data from each day of the calendar year to determine the impact of each of these factors on my pain levels (BASDAI score), including the interaction between effects. Sometimes, filtering out the effects from a variety of factors can be difficult in a complex system with many variables. In this type of analysis, randomness is a key part of the analysis, and multiple factors being changed at the same time can be accounted for, although I was still only dealing with six general categories. In this chart, a larger number is bad; it increases my pain/stiffness score on the BASDAI scale.

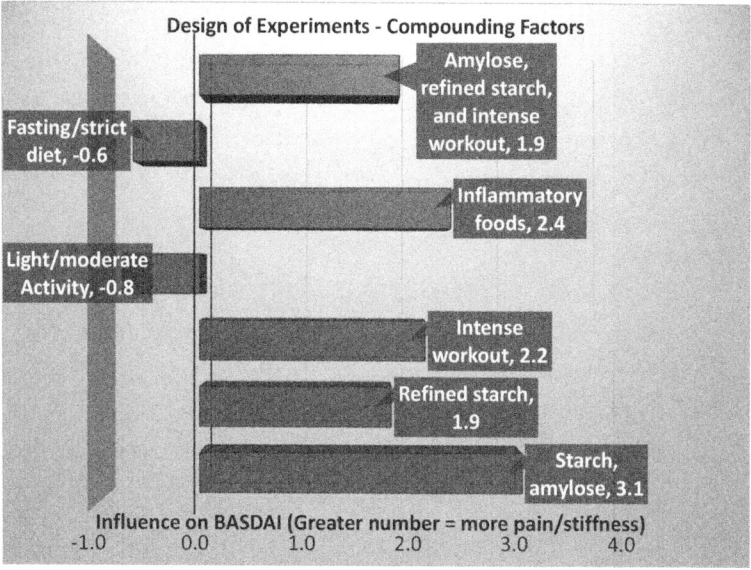

The analysis revealed some interesting information, that was not apparent at first but upon review, fit the data. Amylose starch on its own seemed to be the biggest single contributing factor. "Intense workout," unfortunately, was another. I suppose I pushed myself too hard, too often, and injury or soreness from a workout, while good on its own if done safely, seemed to contribute to arthritis pain as well. Going through my notes, I found it was intense resistance training that most often triggered flare-ups, and in those instances, strict diet on its own was not enough to prevent the flare-ups. Moderate activity had the reverse effect, as did maintaining a strict diet with intermittent fasting. In a nutshell, this chart tells us to keep up the moderate activity, and keep a clean diet away from inflammatory foods and starches.

This analysis considers natural factors only; if medication was on this chart, it would have done very well.

## Clear positive benefits

Below is a list of medications, supplements, treatments, and daily activities that I've commented on for effectiveness in my personal management of AS. Through my daily log, over the course of several years, these items have provided my with clear positive benefits in managing pain and stiffness.

Medication:
- Prednisone: Showed immediate relief, but relief seemed to be short-lived and resulted in heart palpitations and other side effects.
- Cortisone shots: Showed immediate local relief the next day and continued relief, with side effect concerns similar to those listed before. In most cases, it was an immediate relief in swelling, followed by a relief in pain and increase in movement. In my last shot (once I was off other medications and about two years into the disease), I received one last cortisone shot in my RH second toe, where I had some synovitis and ongoing swelling. The swelling immediately went down, but the shot didn't resolve the root cause of the issue at all. Mobility improved, pain was lessened but persisted and the foot was sensitive to pressure. Fixing shoe problems (flat shoes, bigger toe box) and avoiding overuse was the long-term solution here.
- Naproxen: Showed moderate sustained benefit. Trying to cut naproxen usually resulted in an increase in pain within six days. Taking it again on tough days provides good improvement, usually the next morning.

Diet:

- Long-term water fasting: two days of fasting typically clears all symptoms. Six-day water fast showed continued improvement, including foot, neck and back pain. Very effective in reducing swelling/warmth/redness, moderate to good effectiveness in reducing pain; however fasting does not resolve stiffness, need to keep daily stretching!
- Omega-3 (DHA): Two capsules with a meal seemed to show relief in a 30-minute time frame and seemed to offer protection from evening soreness setting in. Benefit required taking these on a regular basis for over a month.
- Kefir: Reintroduced kefir after week-long work conference. This seemed to be the only change that led to a gradual recovery in my back (scale five to scale zero) over a period of eight days.
- Intermittent fasting: Showed immediate relief the next day, and continued relief (so far as long as intermittent fasting is continued). I seem to feel the most of this benefit in the morning, once I start getting hungry (fast usually for 16 hours but benefits begun to be felt at 13–15 hours of fast). Extending this fasting till noon (18 hours) shows even more benefit.
- Periodic fasting: Three-day water fast showed total resolution of remaining soreness in feet on second and third day. Muscle soreness and fatigue cleared up completely, without glycine. (Note, I also took a break from biking during this time, and that may have contributed to giving my muscles a rest). Another three-and-a-half-day fast showed total resolution of all symptoms, including neck gland soreness, best fasting experience so far. I didn't have a single three-day fast that didn't show good results.
- Long-term IF, 20:4, on a regular basis, gives me good energy, (no fatigue), keeps me strong on the bike and light feeling throughout the day, and gives me a chance to have

a nice big meal in the evening without guilt, bloating, or any flare-ups (observing the no-starch rule and sticking to healthy foods and avoiding overeating past a full feeling). Occasional, typical mild hunger pangs but I would describe the fast period as comforting and a relief from food.
- Calorie restriction: Period through January and February 2018 showed lots of 100% days when I was counting calories and restricting calories to 1900 cal/day on average (I had some feast and fast days in there as well, not 1900cal/day).
- Magnesium: Resolved constipation perfectly during extended water fast within 12hours. Also reduced muscle soreness in same time frame. Also try magnesium salts for muscles.

Physical:
- Posture: Daily focus on straight back posture and core support has helped back considerably over a period of four days. Mid-back stiffness was reduced by going back to a straight posture.
- Stretching: Physio exercises and Pilates shows good progression in range of motion and freedom from pain in back especially. Foot stretches and exercise shows a quick benefit for plantar fasciitis symptoms.
- Movement/exercise: Stretching feet in bed before standing helps greatly with reduction in pain in morning. Occasional walking helps with foot and back stiffness at work and at home. Movement with chores (cleaning, garden work, light renovations) at home helps greatly, as long as I'm not on my feet for an extended period. If I have a day with steady, light/moderate activity, I can go the entire day without noticing any pain. Intense aerobic activity (sprinting on the bike), as long as there is no major impact or strain to joints, gives a "runner's high" and totally clears up any pain.

- Padding: For plantar fasciitis, arch supports plus thick socks in shoes, or thick socks in my slippers at home give cushioning and avoid heel pain in the evening. Careful shoes are not too tight, or it can make the pain in the toes worse.
- Rest: A general RICE (Rest, Ice, Compression, Elevation) strategy was effective in bringing down inflammation and pain in peripheral arthritis in my RH ball of foot. Taking a three-week break from cycling was actually more effective in resolving the issue than the cortisone shot I received a month earlier. However, this area of pain seemed to be more related to repetitive use injury than it was arthritis. Initially pain increased with rest, but after about two weeks, pain and swelling cleared.

## *Moderate positive benefits*

In my daily log, these items have provided me with moderate positive benefits. The benefit in managing pain and stiffness was either mild or not always consistent, but I list them here because they may work better for you.

Diet
- Removing/substituting cereal, bread, pasta, a reduced complex carb intake. I made a conscious effort to reduce carbs and felt benefit soon after. Sufficient fat or simple carbs (natural glucose or fructose) in the diet keeps fatigue at bay. Low-RS foods (Naan bread) seem tolerable, but not beneficial, so if you want some breads in your diet they need to be in moderation. After trialling and tolerating some cereals and breads for testing, I removed these from my diet again and felt an improvement (scale one to two to scale zero).

- Diet #3: Keto diet broke the recovery plateau and seemed to be reducing pain and increasing energy further. Lean diet (no overeating) and strict avoidance of carbs and sugar seemed to help after a couple days (noticed after a weekend of bad eating). Now I'm noticing this is not the very low carbs, but very low complex carbs (starches, polysaccharides) that seems to be helping. Now I'm finding that it is specifically resistant starch (amylose) while I can tolerate some RDS (amylopectin) but this should still be in moderation.
- Cat's claw: Two capsules seem to consistently give short-term (24-hour) relief. One capsule before bed has a moderate reduction with overnight stiffness and cramping.
- Gelatin: Had a gelatin serving, plus two bowls of chicken-feet soup, plus a plate of chicken feet, and slept better than I have in a couple weeks, with less pain, stiffness or cramping. Seems to have a mild effect and I need to consume a decent quantity to notice any benefit.
- Brussels sprouts on a number of occasions seemed to give me decent benefit. While they usually caused flatulence a few hours after a dinner meal, they repeatedly seemed to support my bowel health and movements and eased swelling pressure at my joints.
- Water before bed reduces muscle cramping and general stiffness overnight. I'm up to use the washroom a couple times anyway and drinking water doesn't change that.
- Waiting till I'm hungry before starting my next meal helps keep a light digestive load and seems to give my body a chance to flush things through.
- Diet strategy #2 (moderate carbs, eating mostly fruit and kefir for first meal of the day) seemed to give better pain improvement and less fatigue over a period of a week than diet strategy #1 (very low carbs) which tends to cause more fatigue, unless you're very consistent with a keto diet. The

very low-carb diet feels therapeutic for short term, but in the long term I feel better on moderate carbs.
- Fruit, kefir, egg and veggies all seem safe after a flare-up and allow a recovery.
- Rest days seem to help with plantar fasciitis and leg muscle soreness/fatigue. Don't overdo it with exercise!
- Fasting: One-day water/coffee fast. This helped reduce symptoms but not as much benefit as the three-day fast. Still ended with mild overnight foot pain and muscle stiffness.

Physical
- Icing: Acute, local pain/swelling relief. Relief is short-lived.
- Heat: Loosens and soothes joint (back, feet) but relief is usually short-lived.

Medication
- Sulfasalazine: Slow response but this seemed to begin helping after three months. I felt improvement when going from four tablets to six per day. However once naproxen was cut (while still taking sulfasalazine), pain returned to feet, back, wrist, which the sulfasalazine was supposed to protect against. It seemed like majority of the benefit was actually from the naproxen. Being stricter on diet helped here. When I discontinued sulfasalazine over a year later, it took another three-and-a-half months to notice an increase in the number of flares in the feet, so it seems the sulfasalazine was protecting against this.

## *Benefits Unknown/unclear*

This list of items didn't provide me with any noticeable benefit in managing pain or stiffness, but there are studies that support them as being beneficial, so certainly you can try them in your case.

There are also items, like the consumption of sufficient glycine in the diet, that may not be noticeable unless observed for a period of several years. If I was glycine deficient for years, how different would I feel? These factors can be very difficult to measure.

Diet
- Curcumin: No benefit noticed.
- Diet #2: Garlic (allicin to suppress HLA-B27) and/or rosemary (ursolic acid to suppress IL-17) seem to show moderate benefit but not clear and difficult to measure/isolate the benefit.
- Glycine: The timing of starting these supplements corresponded to the time when I tried cutting naproxen. Before then, I was unable to cut out naproxen for more than a few days at a time. Glycine increased to 10–12 g/d seems to have a corresponding improvement in pain reduction and extends the number of days I don't need naproxen. Glycine before bed seems to make me very thirsty. When cutting out regular glycine, I noticed increased pain in calves the next day, for four days, despite no changes to biking routine. When I reintroduced gelatin, calf soreness seems down the next morning. I restarted with a magnesium glycine supplement in January 2018 and noticed a clear improvement in sleep and reduction in overnight muscle tension in both my legs and shoulders. No direct impact on the arthritis was noticed but this is a supplement that helps indirectly. (Blancas-Flores G1, 2012), (Zhong Z1, 2003), (Herron, 2015).
- Once I was in the habit of avoiding sugars and starches, higher-GI food (like sticky white rice and raisins), I got flushed in the face, warm, almost like after a couple alcoholic drinks. It never seemed to have a direct impact on arthritis flare-ups, but I generally don't like the feeling as it felt inflammatory and seemed to be just another incentive to stay away from high-GI foods.

## GENERAL MANAGEMENT AND SOLUTIONS

Physical
- Periodical resting of feet, still and without movement, may help with recovery. I had a few instances, such as resting my feet during a train ride and during a meeting, where I swear I could literally feel my joints healing. It was almost a throbbing sensation, not painful, but resulted in less pain, and that lasted for 15 minutes or so. For my left heel, careful stretching without snapping the joint also seemed to help with recovery.

*Clear negative effects*

Maybe some of these are obvious, but this is a list of some factors I've noticed that clearly made my arthritis worse.

Physical
- Physical impact to joints (tennis, running).
- Posture at work and prolonged time in awkward postures.
- Extended inactivity, especially when constrained sitting (like in a car for over half-an-hour) or sitting still at work (one hour) causes acute soreness in feet and lower back. As my symptoms came under control, I could sit longer in the car, but still usually not much more than an hour. A lazy weekend without any intensive activity shows a gradual daily increase in foot pain.
- Consistent pressure on feet cause numbness. I've noticed this on long bike rides, and finally realized it when sitting at work with pressure against the balls of my feet while sitting. Being stationary on my feet for a longer period of time also causes this, and I found I need to alternate with sitting/walking.
- Shoes that are too tight. In some occasions, wearing thick socks provides extra cushioning, but compression made the

right ball of my foot much worse. Immediate relief with thinner socks and a sufficiently large shoe box.
- Overactivity causing overnight cramping. I was feeling 100% for a week then did some hard biking and walking and noticed cramping in calves the next night and an increase in general foot stiffness, despite taking glycine.
- Physical exertion on the bike—several hard rides—seems to aggravate the plantar fasciitis in the left heel and also causes toe pain. Usually when I ride hard, I'm pressing hard on the balls of my feet. Pedalling/standing for a couple days highly aggravated my right heel.

Diet
- Overeating generally results in gas, general swelling and sometimes flare-up. Heavy digestive load feels like it results in undigested carbs and may be just as bad as starches.
- A "binge day" of eating will cause a flare-up and/or a couple days of inflammation. Overeating in general seems to contribute to flare-up.
- Carbs. During camping, I had pizza for the first time in a long time, and too many pistachios and almonds, and turkey sausages high in omega-6, and I had a very significant flare in feet and minor back flare-up within a few hours. Pistachios are also very high in omega-6 but I don't expect this to have caused the immediate effect that it did.
- Processed meats, like Korean BBQ (possibly MSG?), turkey sausage, BBQ chicken sausage (dark meat, high omega-6), also cooked on high heat. This was the only change in diet that could explain big flare-up in feet soon after.
- Omega-6: peanut butter and almond butter repeatedly cause flare-ups.
- Commercial foods and most restaurant foods with added sauces—I later determined this was starch content in sauce.

## GENERAL MANAGEMENT AND SOLUTIONS

- Synthetic sugary foods, like the trail mix with cranberry and "yogurt" (mostly sugar at 19 g/serving) or cheap ice cream with additives (Polysorbate 80 and carboxymethylcellulose, both inflammatory). I have an energy spike from the sugar, but a noticeable crash, and with the crash comes increased pain and major fatigue. Natural sweet fruit like apples, raisins, berries and honey is no problem; however, milk chocolate in excess (due to sugar content?) has caused a clear flare in the feet.
- Starch. At a point I tried to add flour back into the diet. This was tolerated to some extent, I believe because the flour had added amylase to help break down amylose starch, but on the second day, heel soreness started to increase and redness and swelling across the toes especially the second toe, which started to show dactylitis for the first time in months. On the third day, I continued the starch and added yeast (homemade bread) and this caused major bloating, heel pain, and minor swelling in feet (March 4). Had a small slice of cake and corn squares (cereal) and had significant right foot pain and moderate swelling that evening and next morning.
- Foods with resistant starch (cashews) seem to also contribute to flare-up. Foods low in amylose (naan bread) not causing a problem.
- Sugar. After a four-day fast and maintaining pretty decent keto diet for a while, I had two pieces of cheesecake during camping. My energy afterwards crashed hard and had a moderate flare-up in my RH heel, about one hour afterwards, that lasted maybe two hours.

Stress
- Acute stress. For example, worrying about my youngest child running off or in danger, I could feel foot pain rising.

Other trends
- Weekends: My log shows a clear trend of flare-ups happening on weekends. Clearly shows there is a lifestyle contribution to AS flare-ups. I would attribute this to too much eating, higher stress, and not enough activity.
- I tend to have the most foot pain when I'm full, bloated or gassy. Definitely a correlation to overeating, even safe foods.

## Suspected cause of my AS

While working on my research, I came to the conclusion that there were three main factors that came together to trigger my arthritis; *Klebsiella*, HLA-B27, and a high starch and omega-6 diet. The onset of my AS was explosive; one week I was 100% my usual self. During a trip overseas, I became sick, with fever, gastrointestinal illness, and less than a week later, severe joint inflammation, starting with my back, came on hard and fast. The first factor I suspect, was a bacterial infection, likely *Klebsiella* bacteria in my gut, and/or Epstein-Barr virus. This would not have caused the AS on its own, except that I later found that I carry a gene called HLA-B27, and there is much research that shows molecular mimicry between the gene and *Klebsiella*, meaning the body confuses itself with the bacteria, and attacks both, causing the inflammation. (Nicholas J Sheehan, The ramifications of HLA-B27, 2004) Looking back, I also was in an eating pattern with a diet that was high in starch, which could allow the *Klebsiella* to proliferate, and a highly inflammatory diet, including high-GI foods and high omega-6 content, which also promoted the inflammation. All these factors were aligned in my life to produce the "perfect storm" of factors, allowing the onset of the disease.

*Klebsiella pneumoniae*, along with *E. Coli* and *Klebsiella oxytoca* are common and typically produce mild to severe illness. They normally enter the body orally and can be found in food.

(Wikipedia, 2018) This is consistent with my case, as I suffered from a major gastrointestinal infection at the onset of my condition. With regards to AS specifically, studies show a very clear link to *Klebsiella* alone. (Ebringer A., 1992) In the case of reactive arthritis, other bacteria including *Salmonella*, *Shigella*, *Yersinia*, *Campylobacter*, *Chlamydia*, *Mycobacterium* and *Brucella* are all suspect, with HLA-B27 shown to enhance the invasion of *Salmonella* into the body, and evidence of bacteria fragments of *Chlamydia*, *Yersinia* and *Salmonella* in the joints of patients. (Nicholas J Sheehan, The ramifications of HLA-B27, 2004). In my personal situation, I was tested for *Chlamydia* during the onset of my symptoms, as one of the routine blood tests. Test results were negative, however it noteworthy that *Klebsiella* is a Gram-negative bacteria, like *Chlamydia*. (Wikipedia, 2018).

Much research has shown molecular mimicry between HLA-B27 and two *Klebsiella* surface molecules as the cause of ankylosing spondylitis as well as patients with AS showed higher levels of anti-*Klebsiella* IgA antibodies, that were correlated to CRP levels. (Collado A1, 1994) Again, this is consistent with my high-CRP blood test results.

In fact, the molecular mimicry between HLA-B27 and *Klebsiella* has been narrowed down to the similarity of just six amino acids. (Nicholas J Sheehan, The ramifications of HLA-B27, 2004). Other research also indicates a mechanism for the antibodies in an HLA-B27 positive individual to "accidentally" bind to HLA-B27. The pathway of the body attacking itself is the concept behind an autoimmune disease such as AS. (Chris Kresser, 2019)

The great work conducted by Dr. Alan Ebringer, and his ground-laying work on the link between AS and *Klebsiella* has been a great guide in my personal effort to reduce symptoms. Some of his findings also indicate that it is not necessarily one infection

*Klebsiella*, but repeated episodes, that can cause recurring flares or allow the disease to go through cycles of inactivity and activity. There is obviously much overlap with symptoms, especially between AS, reactive arthritis and psoriatic arthritis, and he goes so far to call "*Klebsiella*-reactive arthritis" a precursor stage in the early and active phases of AS. (Ebringer A., The relationship between Klebsiella infection and ankylosing spondylitis., 1989)

Again, this is consistent with my case, as I suffered from repeated gastrointestinal infections in the years leading up to the onset of my condition, usually coinciding with international travel. I have to admit excessive drinking and eating often also coincided.

## Causes – root cause and corrective action

What do I think is the cause of AS? It's the body's autoimmune response to an infection, a bacterial infection, caused by *Klebsiella* and/or similar virus like Epstein-Barr virus. An injured, porous gut lining allows the bacteria to enter the body through the gut lining, and the reaction with HLA-B27 causes autoimmune responses in the form or arthritis, much like a flu might cause body aches. If we could physically see the intestine, scraped, infected and bleeding, we could understand how this infection could happen through the gut. We could see how eating inflammatory foods could worsen the condition. We could see how starch, feeding the bacteria and allowing it to proliferate on an infected wound, could worsen the symptoms, continue the infection, and contribute to gastrointestinal problems.

In this light, all the solutions listed can be clearly seen as solutions to the problem. When the source of AS is viewed as a bacterial infection on a wounded intestine, it's easier to see how something like apple cider vinegar might clean the gut like hydrogen peroxide might clear a topical wound. This general concept seems to fit all

## GENERAL MANAGEMENT AND SOLUTIONS

my observations with how the disease behaves and reacts to my activity, diet and eating pattern.

Likely process of AS progression:

1. HLA-B27 is present.
2. Lesions in colon are present due to inflammatory diet and/or overeating. An inflammatory diet, oxidative stress or lifestyle may increase TNFα, which has been shown to cause mucosal dysfunction in the colon, producing an opening of tight junctions.
3. *Klebsiella* is present in colon due to infection. Note this may also be EBV, *Salmonella* or another bacteria as the trigger.
4. *Klebsiella* spreads due to high-amylose diet.
5. Bacteria passes through colon through lesions.
6. Body reacts to bacteria in body with antibodies.
7. Autoimmune process begins when antibodies attack HLA-B27, explained by biomimicry.
8. Autoimmune process becomes independent of continuous exposure to the initial environmental trigger, however, once learned, the adaptive immune response may be triggered by the detection of Klebsiella in the colon through what are called "Toll-Like Receptors."

Symptoms need to be managed as well. Since AS ultimately expresses itself through joint inflammation, then physiotherapy, stretching, exercises, anti-inflammatory foods all need to be considered to prevent the inflammation that leads to bone growth and bamboo spine, and allow for the healing of entheses. But these are all symptoms. The gut needs to be healed and the bacteria need to be eradicated. Intermittent fasting needs to be incorporated to give rest time for the gastrointestinal system, giving it opportunity to heal, and not re-aggravating it with inflammatory, processed or chemical-laden foods.

In engineering we commonly use a tool called *Root Cause and Corrective Action Analysis* (RCCA). It's generally used in a production environment to investigate the reasons a product failed, to identify all the contributing causes, and to apply solutions to correct all contributors to avoid the problem occurring again. It assumes that each cause has a contributing action and condition, and it requires asking "why" multiple times until the root of the problem is uncovered. You can continue to ask why until the answer becomes ridiculous, and that's when you know you've asked enough times. For example, why did the airbag not deploy in the event of an accident? A wire was not connected properly. Why was it not connected? There were no in process checks. The operator was not aware of the procedure. There was no testing completed. The procedure was not clear. These would all be areas that need to be addressed. But dig deeper. Is the training procedure lacking? Are new employees not trained to the requirements? Are documents not updated on a regular basis? New levels of questioning will reveal deeper problems and applying solutions to all potential issues will make a robust production system, and ensure we make a good product, with the goal to make it right every time.

This was my approach to managing AS. I identified as many causes as I could, applied solutions to as many of them as possible, trying to take a holistic approach. Maybe some of these were possible contributors, maybe not all proven, but addressing all that I could would provide a high certainty that I would resolve the problem. Some contributing causes can't be changed. I can't change the fact that I have the HLA-B27 gene and that's a contributing cause, so, I don't worry about it, and instead I focus my energy on all the other factors in my life I *can* change. I encourage you to take the same approach in your situation.

# GENERAL MANGEMENT AND SOLUTIONS

**Root Cause and Corrective Action,**
1. Definition of the problem
2. Determine relationships between causes
3. Identify effective solutions
4. Implement and track solutions

Cause and Effect. Each effect has at least two causes in the form of actions and conditions. Actions shown in grey, conditions and solutions shown in white.

| | | | | |
|---|---|---|---|---|
| Ankylosing Spondylitis | Autoimmune response | HLA-B27 | Genetics | |
| | | Bacterial infection | Probiotics | |
| | | AND/OR | | |
| | | HLA-B27 | | |
| | | EBV Infection | Probiotics | |
| | | Re-activation of latent EBV Infection | Fasting | |
| | | AND/OR | | |
| | | HLA-B27 | | |
| | | Klebsiella | Probiotics | |
| | | | Oil of Thyme | |
| | | | Oil of Oregano | |
| | | AND | | |
| | | High starch diet | Low Starch Diet | |
| | Joint inflammation | Klebsiella | | |
| | | Intestinal inflammation, leaky gut syndrome | Free Radicals | Antioxidants |
| | | | Proinflammatory Cytokines | |
| | Sacroiliac Joint, back, neck, uveitis | | TNF-a | Diet, Natural TNF-a antagonists |
| | | Inflammatory diet, high Omega-6 | Processed, packaged foods | Diet, fresh whole foods |
| | | | Overeating | Calorie restriction |
| | | | High Sugar diet | Diet, Keto, ketone bodies |
| | | | High omega-6 foods | Omega-3 ALA |
| | Fatigue | Iron deficiency | Diet, fresh whole foods | |
| | | Metabolic issues | Calorie restriction | |

| | | | | |
|---|---|---|---|---|
| **Comorbidities** | Diverticulosis | Inflamed joints and/or bowel | Fasting | |
| | | Genetics | | |
| | | Inflamed joints and/or bowel | Proinflammatory Cytokines | Parasympathetic nervous system (rest and digest) |
| | | Emotional factors | Sympathetic nervous system (fight and flight) | Stress management |
| | Achilles Tendonitis | Excessive physical Stress, insufficient rest | Adequate rest, alternating activities | |
| | | Inflammatory diet | | |
| | Capsulitis | Excessive physical Stress, insufficient rest | Adequate rest, alternating activities | |
| | | Flat feet | Weak muscles | Exercises |
| | | Pronounced second toe | Excessive physical Stress, insufficient rest | Adequate rest, alternating activities |
| | Enthesis | Excessive physical Stress, insufficient rest | Adequate rest, alternating activities | |
| | Temporo-mandibular disorder | Excessive physical Stress, insufficient rest | Adequate rest, alternating activities | |

This table summarizes my strategy. Each condition (orange), and action (blue), needed a solution (green). What is the solution to the condition of having the HLA-B27 gene? There may not always be a solution. But if the associated action, for example, a bacterial infection, has a solution applied that will prevent it from occurring, then the HLA-B27 will not surface as a problem.

## Health strategy

In this section I would like to summarize the importance of diet, medication, physiotherapy, exercise, stress management, and in general the importance of the holistic approach that was important in my AS recovery. During my recovery I set a number of goals for myself and constantly adjusted the actions that I felt I needed to accomplish to achieve my goals.

### General diet strategy

- Moderate carbs (lots of vegetables, carbs from flax or chia plus simple sugars from fruits and veggies). Avoid resistant starch entirely, anything that tests black.
- Moderate protein (still allow for some fish or egg or dairy, omega-3s).
- Rely on intermittent fasting or fasting days for ketogenesis.
- Lower calorie consumption in general.

### Specific goals

- Disease (infection) remission: low-starch diet, sulfasalazine, and build/maintain gut flora.
- Reducing inflammation: omegas, IF, mind and spirit, and sulfasalazine.
- Joint repair/healing: hydration, bone broth (gelatin/collagen), and physiotherapy.

- Pain relief: icing/heat, medication, cat's claw for back flare-ups, and IF.
- Mobility: exercise and stretching.
- Replace medication with supplements and replace supplements with diet.

## Specific targets

I then established some more specific future targets to aim for, and assessed their effectiveness in my daily log as I made progress:

- Use glycine with magnesium 10 g/d to reduce muscle cramping associated with exercise/fasting.
- Reduce omega-3 supplement if getting enough from fish. Reduce omega-3 requirements by reducing omega-6 intake (maintain an omega-6:3 intake balance closer to 1:1).
- Reduce animal protein, and add additional sources of veggie protein and fibre.
- Phase out iron supplement if getting enough from fish/seafood/raisins/liver. Occasional liver in the diet once a week seemed to help keep iron levels up and fatigue at bay.
- Reduce non-healthy fats from diet (high inflammatory omega-6s, trans fats).
- Reduce breads and cereals to one small serving per day max, non-amylose or eliminate entirely if you're comfortable with it. Phase out amylose completely.
- Increase high antioxidant fruits. While sugar should be minimized, don't avoid healthy fruits that also provide fibre and antioxidants (pomegranate and golden berries, blueberries, raspberries, and apple skins). Focus on berries and other low-GI fruit.
- Eliminate dependence on naproxen.
- Replace glycine with gelatin in diet.

- Increasing fruits to increase non-digestible fibres like cellulose and lignin.

In addition to this, I have incorporated the strategies I've outlined in chapter 6 (fasting) chapters 7 and 8 (diet), chapter 9 (exercise and stress management).

*Closing recommendations*

Summary of actions required for reversal of autoimmune response:

1. Specific to AS, a low-amylose diet needs to be implemented to reduce *Klebsiella* numbers in the colon. A reduction in starch on its own has also been shown to reduce serum IgA.
2. In the case of infection such as EBV, which may have triggered to autoimmune response, the infection needs to be halted. If medication, including antibiotics, is recommended in your case to address such an infection, so be it.
3. A transition to natural, anti-inflammatory corrections are required to calm the response in the body.
4. The use of fasting as a therapeutic tool is required for anti-inflammatory benefit and to reduce the autoimmune response and to allow the body and colon to heal and repair.
5. Small intestinal bacterial overgrowth (SIBO) diet or similar low-fermentation diet will assist in colon recovery. Start with the recommendations provided and use the elimination diet to customize your diet to your lifestyle and needs.
6. Since HLA-B27 levels or other genetic factors cannot be reduced, a reduction in triggering factors such as *Klebsiella* must be eliminated, and anti-inflammatory measures including food, fasting, medication, and icing are required to reduce the autoimmune response.

Once stability is achieved, a moderate maintenance program can be used:

1. Once the body reduces the autoimmune response and colon recovery has progressed, starch becomes more tolerated by the patient and the disease enters a dormant or low-activity phase.
2. Occasional intermittent fasting is recommended to maintain colon health.
3. SIBO is recommended to maintain colon health.
4. The maintenance of a low-starch diet is recommended to prevent re-proliferation of *Klebsiella*.
5. The maintenance of anti-inflammatory foods and lifestyle is recommended to keep the autoimmune response in the body low, since sufficient inflammation alone may restart the autoimmune response against HLA-B27.
6. The risk of re-infection by *Klebsiella* or food-borne bacteria (e.g., *Shigella*, *Salmonella*, *Yersinia*) or viral infection should be reduced as much as possible through sanitary environment and practices.
7. Foods that promote healthy gut bacteria that can supplant *Klebsiella* should be maintained.

I've been told many times that there is no cure for AS. A "cure" means a patient no longer has a particular condition anymore. Diseases with no cure like AS and other forms of arthritis, fortunately, have medical treatments that can help manage the disease. I've found through my experience that treatments to manage the disease can be natural as well. As for a cure? I remain cautiously optimistic; only time will tell.

# CHAPTER 11

# RECIPES

I would be doing you a disservice if I did not include some information on some recipes. If anything positive has come out of my experience with AS (besides, hopefully, this book), it would be the knowledge I've gained surrounding food, diet and recipes. A few years ago, I only knew a few basic recipes, but having to cook foods from scratch, using basic ingredients, taught me many things about the food we eat, and how to make it nutrient-dense, low-starch, anti-inflammatory, and generally healthy. These are a few of my favourite recipes that have served me well throughout the past few years. Make note of the benefits they provide to managing arthritis and adapt them to your own dietary preferences.

## Starch-free meal ideas

*Breakfast*

*Probiotic Oatmeal Substitute*

Serves 1

Ingredients:
- 250 ml (1 cup) kefir
- 45 ml (3 Tbsp) ground flax (optional, see cautions)
- 15 ml (1 Tbsp) hemp hearts (unground)
- 15 ml (1 Tbsp) chia (soaked, optional) and/or coconut flour (optional)
- Add fruits like strawberries
- Optional to add ricotta, cinnamon and nutmeg to taste. Dip with cauliflower!

Directions:
Pre-soak chia with approximately 250 ml (1 cup) of water. Mix immediately and continuously to prevent chia from clumping, until the chia begins to gelatinize. Hand-blend all ingredients and top with fruit.

Benefits:
A good quality kefir will contain probiotics that are good for digestive health. Flax contains omega-3 ALA oils that are beneficial for colon health. All ingredients make this a low-sugar, ketogenic option.

Cautions:
Flax is high in lignans, a type of phytoestrogen that can cause estrogenic effects in the body. If you are a man, I would recommend limiting your intake. I twice developed a swelling behind the nipple (diagnosed by my doctor as gynecomastia) that I was able to clear up by a change in diet.

## Coconut Cheese Yogurt

Serves 1

Ingredients:
- 30 ml (2 Tbsp) raisins
- 30 ml (2 Tbsp) hemp
- 56 ml (2 heaping Tbsp) coconut flour
- 250 ml (1 cup) kefir or other milk of choice
- Optional to add mascarpone cheese or 30 ml (2 Tbsp) ricotta cheese. For a lower-carb version, substitute some of the coconut flour with flax flour and remove raisins.

Directions:
Mix and serve!

Benefits:
Use a good quality kefir if possible for a healthy dose of probiotics. Coconut flour is low-carb and adds a pleasant thickness and texture to the yogurt. Hemp provides some healthy GLA oils.

## Chia Bowl

Serves 4

Ingredients:
- 125 ml (½ cup) chia
- 375 ml (1.5 cups) water
- 250 ml (1 cup) kefir, almond milk or other milk of choice
- Optional to add whipped cream and fruit like blueberries and strawberries
- Optional to add hemp or whole nuts

Directions:
Whisk chia in water to gelatinize chia, then add almond milk. Top with fruit, whip cream, hemp and nuts.

## Cauliflower and Zucchini Omelette

Serves 6

Ingredients:
- 300 g (approximately ½ head) cauliflower
- 1 medium zucchini
- 1 broccoli crown
- 5 eggs
- Salt, pepper
- Toppings including Havarti cheese, diced avocado, olives

Directions:
Grate cauliflower, zucchini and broccoli into a mixing bowl. Beat in eggs and add salt and pepper to taste. Cook on medium-low heat until egg sets fully through.

Benefits:
This is enough for the whole family. Cauliflower is a great filler and it's hard to tell how little egg is in there compared to a typical omelette. Using the cauliflower also makes it low-sugar/carb and keto friendly.

## Cauliflower and Spinach Omelette

Serves 6

Ingredients:
- 300 g or ½ cauliflower head
- 250 g or 1 bunch fresh spinach, chopped
- 1 medium zucchini
- 5 eggs
- 1 or 2 bell peppers
- ½ large onion
- ½ head broccoli
- ½ bunch of asparagus
- Top with cheese

Directions:
Dice and steam the onion first for about 7–10 minutes. Dice and add in the peppers, broccoli and asparagus and continue steaming for another 5 minutes. While steaming, grate the cauliflower, zucchini and chop the spinach. Allow steamed ingredients to cool and mix in with grated veggies, then beat in eggs. Add a pinch of salt and pepper to taste and fry or bake on medium-low for approximately 20 minutes. Use a healthy oil with a high smoke point like ghee or avocado oil. Top with sharp cheddar or a cheese of your choice.

Benefits:
All those veggies are good for you. Antioxidants from zucchini, suppressing NF-kB through broccoli, and sulfur from cauliflower to help your body produce glutathione.

## Cauliflower Hash Browns

Serves 6

Ingredients:
- 500 g cauliflower
- 3 eggs
- 1 bunch green onion, 1 zucchini or other veggies to taste
- Salt and pepper to taste

Directions:
Grate cauliflower, spread on baking sheet and bake on low heat at 250°F for 30–40 minutes to dry the cauliflower, stirring every 10 minutes or so. Allow to cool and stir in grated zucchini and chopped green onion in a bowl. Add salt and pepper. Beat in eggs. On a good quality, high-heat oil like coconut oil or avocado oil, fry on medium heat by dropping approximately ½-cup dollops on the pan. Fry for approximately 5 minutes and flip, then fry for another 5 minutes.

Benefits:
The cauliflower provides a good source of sulfur, and the oils are healthy for the body as well, and safe to fry with below their smoke point temperature.

## Coconut Wrap

Serves 1

Ingredients:
- 1 coconut wrap*
- 100 g healthy protein such as sardines, herring, or 2 scrambled eggs
- 1 Tbsp kefir or low-sugar yogurt
- Add fruit (diced apple, pomegranate, berries)

* If you can find coconut wraps in your area, I highly recommend them. They are typically made from coconut meat, curry powder and salt and are certified organic. They make a great tortilla substitute.

Directions:
Lightly blend the fish with kefir and apply to the wrap. Top with fruit and wrap. Simple!

Benefits:
Always choose a good quality source of complete proteins that comes naturally packaged in a food with healthy oils that your body needs anyway.

## Salads/snacks, lunches

### Purple Cabbage Salad

Serves 2

Ingredients:
- ¼ head purple cabbage
- ½ medium sized onion (red or white)
- 1 bell pepper, red, orange or yellow
- 500 ml (2 cups) washed and chopped white mushrooms (approximately measured)
- 1 Tbsp coconut oil
- 175 g black olives
- Salt and pepper to taste
- Lightly fried herring or salmon, with skin on (optional)

Directions: Wash and chop all ingredients. Both the onions and mushrooms can be lightly sautéed in a little bit of coconut oil on medium heat. Another healthier option would be to steam these with the other ingredients. Start by steaming the cabbage, onions, and mushrooms till moderately soft (about 5–7 minutes), then add in the peppers for the last 5 minutes since they require less steaming time. Transfer to plate and add uncooked, chopped black olives and top with some additional coconut oil, salt and pepper. The flavour of the olives and coconut oil blend nicely together and provide a filling, satisfying meal.

Benefits:
The oleocanthal from the olives are anti-inflammatory and the onion provides a healthy dose of quercetin. For extra anti-arthritis benefit, add in some lightly fried fish with the skin on. The cabbage contains proline, which together with the glycine from the fish skin, helps form collagen to promote joint growth and repair.

## Fish Avocado Dip

Serves 2

Ingredients:
- 1 whole avocado
- 100–200 g of canned sardines, herring, or mackerel
- 3 Tbsp of extra virgin olive oil
- Salt and pepper to taste

Directions:
Cut open avocado in half and remove stone. Dice the avocado and scoop out into a bowl. Remove the fish from the can and mix in with the avocado. Add olive oil, salt and pepper. Mix in well but do not make too smooth; the creamy texture of the avocado balances nicely with the texture of the fish.

Benefits:
This is a simple dip that acts as a superstar to fight arthritis. The oleocanthal from the olive oil, together with the omega-3 oils from the fish are two of the best tools to fight arthritis. The avocado contains monounsaturated fats and MCTs that provide good energy. This is very much a zero-starch and keto dip.

## Coconut Wrap

Serves 3

Ingredients:
- 3 coconut wraps
- 1 fillet baked trout
- 250 ml (1 cup) riced or grated cauliflower
- ¼ head chopped lettuce
- ½ bunch green onion
- 1 medium bell pepper, any colour (orange will be the sweetest)
- ½ diced avocado
- 250 ml (1 cup) chopped fresh spinach

Directions:
Grate cauliflower, spread on a pan and dry in the oven at 200°F for approximately 40 minutes. Mix after 20 minutes to ensure even drying. Fillet the trout, skin on, and bake in the oven at 400°F for approximately 12 minutes. The time will vary depending on the size of your fish, but a nice and small rainbow trout should bake quickly while a thicker fillet of steelhead trout could take around 20 minutes. Season with salt, celery salt, and dill. Allow the trout to cool before placing in the wrap, otherwise the heat from the fish will cause the wrap to sweat coconut oil. Top with the riced cauliflower. Chop the spinach and lightly fry or steam. Chop the remaining ingredients and add to your wrap.

Benefits:
Trout is a wonderful oily fish that contains plenty of the omega-3 oils you need, plus the skin contains amino acids like glycine for joint repair. The coconut wrap is a great zero-starch alternative that contains MCT oils to provide rapidly digested oils. If you suffer from low energy levels due to anemia like I did, this wrap is an iron absorption powerhouse. Spinach delivers the iron, the fish provides B-12, and the bell pepper provides vitamin C, both cofactors in iron absorption. Don't be tempted to add cheese to this wrap or anything containing significant amounts of calcium that can prevent iron absorption.

## Fish Wrap

Serves 1

Ingredients:
- one small fillet of trout or salmon
- 100 g Swiss cheese or similar
- 1 whole avocado, diced
- 50 g sprouts, broccoli
- 1 large red chard leaf or kale leaf

Directions:
Season the fillet with salt and dill and bake on avocado oil at approximately 400°F for 12 minutes (depending on fillet size). Sufficient oil will prevent the skin from burning or sticking to the pan. Steam or blanch the chard leaf or kale leaf gently and briefly and the leaf as a wrap. Place baked trout into leaf and top with grated cheese, avocado and sprouts.

Benefits:
Don't be afraid to use sufficient oil since this is healthy oil with a high smoke point. This is a healthier option for baking anyway since it will prevent charring/blackening of the fish skin, which would otherwise introduce carcinogens. This combination will give a healthy dose of both monounsaturated fats and omega-3 fats. Try substituting the red chard with a coconut wrap for a more traditional wrap, but make sure the fish is cool before placing on the coconut wrap as the heat will cause the coconut wrap to melt and drip oil which will make for messy eating.

Cautions:
Raw kale and chard can be bitter. Kale (and cruciferous vegetables in general) may affect thyroid function in excess. Chard has high levels of an antinutrient called oxalic acid, so I recommend it lightly steamed.

## Fish Galareta (Jelly)

Serves 2

Ingredients:
- 1 pack gelatin (ideally grass-fed bovine gelatin)
- 100 g (1 can) smoked herring in water
- 15 ml (1 Tbsp) olive oil
- 1 hard boiled egg
- ¼ bunch of fresh parsley, diced
- pinch of salt and pepper
- 100 g steamed cabbage or sauerkraut (diced, optional)

Directions:
Mix gelatin with water or vegetable broth per gelatin package, then add all ingredients. Place in fridge for approximately 4 hours until set.

Benefits:
*Galareta* is a traditional Eastern European dish, often made with fish and egg, but often other veggies like carrot and peas. This is my own version, using of course, herring for its high omega-3 content. Cabbage in the mix, together with the glycine from the fish skin and gelatin, provide a synergistic proline/glycine benefit for joint health.

## Cauliflower Salad

Serves 1

Ingredients:
- ¼ head cauliflower, finely chopped
- ¼ bunch of green onions, peppers, lettuce, all chopped
- cottage cheese and sour cream.

Directions:
Chop and mix all ingredients.

Benefits:
A good and simple salad. I love the taste combination between the cauliflower and sour cream. Cauliflower is best in its raw form and is a good source of sulfur which will help synthesize glutathione for antioxidant support.

Cautions:
Be careful with your choice of cottage cheese and sour cream, I've found many in the store to contain corn or potato starch, which should be avoided, and sometimes with a list of other un-necessary additives.

## Shrimp Salad

Serves 2

Ingredients:
- ¼ head minced cauliflower
- 6–8 pieces cooked shrimp or prawns
- ½ avocado
- 125 ml (½ cup) sour cream
- ½ bunch green onion
- 3 sticks celery, chopped
- ¼ bulb finely diced onion
- squirt of lemon juice

Directions:
Dice and mix all ingredients and serve cold.

Benefits:
Another good salad if you're trying to get more sulfur-rich cauliflower in your diet. The shrimp, avocado and sour cream make a nice, rich and creamy combination. Again, be sure you're using good quality sour cream without added starch.

## Tuna Salad

Serves 2

Ingredients:
- 250 ml (approximately 2 cans) canned, light tuna
- 3–4 sticks of celery
- 3–4 dill pickles
- 30 ml (2 Tbsp) mustard
- Pinch of salt and pepper

Directions:
Dice and mix all ingredients and serve cold. Optional to pre-steam the celery to soften it slightly to match the texture of the pickles.

Benefits:
A simple and quick salad that is low-calorie, filling, and moderate protein. I love the combination of mustard and pickle. Mustard has shown to increase IL-10.

## Cauliflower Mash

Serves 4

Ingredients:
- 1 large cauliflower
- ¼ cup cream cheese
- ¼ cup parmesan
- ¼ cup sour cream
- 1 cup grated cheddar
- ½ tsp garlic powder
- ½ tsp salt
- ¼ tsp pepper

Directions:
Boil cauliflower for 15 minutes, drain, blend, top with chopped green onion and remaining ingredients.

Benefits:
If you love your mashed potatoes, you will like this recipe. All the better with a high-sulfur food like cauliflower and allicin from the garlic to suppress HLA-B27.

## *Coleslaw*

Serves 4

Ingredients:
- 1 whole green cabbage
- ¼ cup red cabbage
- ¼ cup onion
- 3 Tbsp lemon juice
- 1 Tbsp apple cider vinegar
- ½ tsp salt and ¼ tsp pepper
- 250 g can full sardines (with skin and bone) in olive oil, or better yet, add your own extra virgin olive oil to ensure you're getting a good quality oil

Directions:
Chop cabbage, drain, add remaining ingredients and blend.

Benefits:
Cabbage providing proline, combined with the glycine from the sardines, again, makes an excellent combination for your joints. Onion adds sulfur and quercetin.

## Soup

Chicken Stock

Serves 8

Ingredients:
- Approximately 500 g chicken feet. Alternatively, use 500 g chicken legs, bone-in
- Non-starchy vegetables like celery, onion, pepper, parsley

Directions:
Rinse chicken feet. Boil hard for 5 minutes, then dump the water, and clean and trim toenails from chicken feet (this is much easier after the 5-minute boil). Place chicken feet in fresh water and boil at lightest setting (simmer) for 2–4 hours with added veggies. If using chicken legs, omit the 5-minute hard boil. The next day, you can change it up and add a can of smoked herring and make it fish soup.

Benefits:
Once you get used to cleaning and working with chicken feet, this can be a great source of gelatin in your diet. It contains so much gelatin that the broth will turn to jelly in the fridge. This acts as a good soup stock that can be used to make cabbage soup by adding shredded red cabbage, fish soup by adding herring, or for use in making galareta.

## Mains

### Crab Cakes

- 1 egg
- 60 ml (¼ cup) mayonnaise
- 30 ml (2 Tbsp) ghee or butter
- Salt, pepper to taste
- 250 g mackerel (if canned with olive oil, include the oil, otherwise drain)
- 500 g crab meat
- 15 ml (1 Tbsp) chives
- 500 ml (2 cups) almond flour

Directions:
Mix and hand-form patties. Aim to have the patties less than 1" thick to ensure they cook through. Fry patties lightly on avocado oil or ghee to brown, then bake at 350°F for 10 minutes per side to cook through.

Benefits:
The arthritis benefits from this recipe will primarily come from the omega-3 oils in the fish. This is a recipe my whole family loves.

Cautions:
The almond flour makes a good wheat flour substitute and is ok in moderation, but don't over-use almond flour if you are battling flares. In moderation it seems ok for me.

## Trout, Whole Baked

Serves 2, depending on fish size

Ingredients:
- Rainbow Trout (whole, cleaned)
- Seasoned salt
- Olive oil

Directions:
Ensure scales are removed from skin. Apply avocado oil in a glass dish and place entire fish in dish. Bake at 400°F for approximately 12 minutes. Check periodically, and when almost cooked, you will be able to separate bones to make fillet. This is my favourite way to fillet a fish since it's less messy, with less chance of missed bones, and no meat is wasted if you fillet it at the right time. Once separated, place the two fillets skin down in the glass dish and broil for a few minutes with seasoned salt. Top with olive oil after cooking. Substitutes could include pan-seared salmon, pan-fried herring, or cooked shrimp. Feel free to top with parsley or other seasoning.

Benefits:
Olive oil provides the oleocanthal and the fish provides the omega-3 oil for anti-inflammatory benefits, while the fish skin provides the collagen for your joints. This is a very simple fish recipe that you can top with dill or lemon to taste, but I love the simple combination of trout with raw olive oil. If you're not typically a seafood lover, do give it a try. Developing a flavour for some of these oily fish to your own liking and making it a regular dish will help your arthritis.

## Pizza - Flax Crust

Serves 4

Ingredients:
- 45 ml (3 Tbsp) ground flax
- 200 ml coconut flour
- 2 eggs
- 30 ml (2 Tbsp) avocado oil
- Oregano or other pizza seasonings, salt

Directions:
Blend dry ingredients first, then add in wet ingredients. Line a pan with wax parchment paper. The coconut flour should dry out the mixture sufficiently to spread out to a flat crust on the paper. Bake at 400°F for approximately 7–12 minutes, depending on thickness of crust. Once dried and baked, top with your choice of sauce and toppings.

Benefits:
One of the few non-wheat crusts that holds together well and is easy to pick up! Flax will provide healthy ALA omega-3 oils, and the coconut flour provides some anti-inflammatory sterols.

## Pizza - Cauliflower Crust

Serves 4

Ingredients:
- 900 g (2 lbs) riced cauliflower, approximately
- 1 egg
- 80 ml (⅓ cup) goat cheese
- 30 ml (2 Tbsp) flax
- Oregano, garlic powder, salt

Directions:
To rice the cauliflower, first grate a full head, then dry in the oven at 200°F for 40–60 minutes, stirring occasionally. Making the cauliflower sufficiently dry will prevent the crust from turning out soggy. It's ok if the cauliflower gets browned in the process. Mix the cauliflower, bake 35 minutes at 400°F. Add topping and re-bake.

Benefits:
In addition to the benefits of cauliflower as described above, the flax seed adds an extra punch of healthy omega-3 ALA oil and a good dose of fibre, both good for colon health, which may be a concern if you have AS.

## Quiche - Egg Salmon

Serves 8

Ingredients:
- 8 eggs
- ½ fillet salmon or steelhead trout
- 350 g ricotta cheese
- 100 g (approximately) fried baby portobello mushrooms
- 400 g lightly steamed and chopped cauliflower
- 300 g lightly steamed and chopped broccoli
- 20 ml (4 tsp) salt

Directions:
In my house, we're constantly making fish, so this recipe assumes you have some leftover baked salmon. The recipe works well with trout or even canned herring or sardines, but the point is to choose something high in omega-3 oils that suites your taste. Start by mixing eggs, ricotta and salt. Add in clumps of diced salmon. Pan fry some diced portobello mushroom, allow to cool and add to the mix. Using ½ a head of cauliflower, grate the cauliflower and broccoli and steam for a few minutes just to soften, allow to cool and add to the mix. Pour the mixture into a pan and bake for 60–75min at 375°F–400°F. Instead of using a pan, this filling can be used with a pie filling such as a flax crust to produce a savoury dinner pie.

Benefits:
The broccoli and cauliflower are both anti-inflammatory and high in sulfur, while the fish provides your omega-3 oils. When selecting eggs, try to use eggs from flax-fed chickens to increase the omega-3 in the egg. While this doesn't really create a high dietary source of omega-3 ALA, it does result in an egg with a lower arachidonic acid omega-6 oil, which is inflammatory. This results in the egg being a much less inflammatory food.

## Portobello With Escargot

Serves 2

Ingredients:
- 2 large portobello mushrooms
- 115 g can of escargot
- 30 ml (2 Tbsp) avocado oil
- 80 ml goat cheese
- ½ fried onion
- 4 cloves garlic
- 60 ml guacamole
- 200 ml red cabbage
- 2 handfuls of fresh spinach

Directions:
Clean and trim portobello mushrooms. Apply avocado oil top and bottom and bake in oven for 10 minutes at 350°F. While the mushrooms are cooking, lightly sauté chopped onion on a frying pan on avocado oil or on water. Remove the mushrooms from the oven and top with canned escargot, onions, diced garlic, and grated red cabbage and cook for another 20 minutes. When cooked, place the mushrooms on a bed of fresh spinach. While hot, top the mushrooms with goat cheese, diced guacamole and serve.

Benefits:
The allicin in garlic, monounsaturated fats from the avocado and sulfur and other benefits from onion and cabbage make this a beneficial meal. With the escargot and goat cheese, you can turn it into an extravagant looking meal for two.

## Rice Substitute

Serves 4

Ingredients:
- 900 g (2 lbs) cauliflower, whole head
- ¼ tsp salt

Directions:
Grate the cauliflower. Bring a pot of water to boil, remove from heat and place cauliflower in hot water for 1–2 minutes to soften. Strain, add salt and mix in.

Benefits:
For those who like rice, this is a very, very simple substitute that is starch-free, low-glycemic index, and provides minerals like sulfur and anti-inflammatory benefits. While sticky white rice is an amylose-free option, I've come to prefer cauliflower prepared in this way.

## Desserts

### Chocolate Squares

Ingredients:
- 75 ml (5 Tbsp) cocoa butter
- 60–75 ml (4–5 Tbsp) cocoa powder
- 25 g stevia
- 75 ml (5 Tbsp) of 100% dark chocolate, if available
- optional raisins and hemp hearts

Directions:
Melt the coconut butter in a pot on low–medium heat. Mix in cocoa powder until dissolved. Add in some dark chocolate to add creaminess, and some stevia to sweeten. Stevia has its own distinct flavour in the recipe, so you may want to opt for honey or maple syrup instead. Pour into forms and allow to cool in freezer. If you can't find cocoa butter, you can substitute with coconut oil, but the end result needs to be refrigerated or it will melt in your hands.

Benefits:
Dark chocolate has anti-inflammatory flavonoids. Sticking to cocoa powder will help you avoid chocolates that are primarily made from sugars and modified milk ingredients. Honey has lots of benefits, including being bactericidal against *Klebsiella*, and maple syrup is a good source of minerals, just make sure it's pure maple syrup and not corn syrup or something blended. Use in moderation due to sugar content. Raisins are also high in sugar so use sparingly.

## Graham Cracker Flax Crust

Serves: Enough for 1 pie crust

Ingredients:
- 200 g flax
- 30 ml (2 Tbsp) ghee
- 15 ml (1 Tbsp) cinnamon
- 60 ml (4 Tbsp) honey (optional)

Directions:
Grind flaxseed finely in a grinder. Mix all ingredients and form by hand into pie shell. This recipe can be eaten raw, or depending on the filling, used it can be baked as well.

Benefits:
The flax is a great source of ALA oils, omega-9s, but use in moderation due to phytoestrogen content. This is a much healthier option for a pie crust than using white refined flour or store-bought pie crusts that contain modified oils or added sugars. The less-processed the better, and if you need to add sugar to cooking, opt for honey or maple syrup and use sparingly.

## Cream Cheese "Icing"

Ingredients:
- 225 g cream cheese (can partially substitute with sour cream or ricotta)
- 125 ml (½ cup) ghee
- 70 g stevia
- 2.5–5ml (½ to 1 tsp) vanilla

Directions:
Cream butter and cream cheese together. Add the sweetener and vanilla extract and beat on high for 2 minutes or until fluffy. As an option, you can use 200 ml of Greek yogurt instead of ghee.

Cautions:
If using yogurt, read the ingredients carefully. They can contain lots of added sugars and starches.

## Buttermilk Ricotta Cheese

Ingredients:
- 6 litres buttermilk
- 1 tsp salt

Directions:
In a large pot, heat buttermilk on low to medium heat, slowly till the curds and whey separate. If buttermilk starts to steam, lower heat. Do not boil. Once curds separate from the whey, add salt, then strain through a cheesecloth. Allow cheese to drain under its own weight and transfer to a container, allow to cool before serving.

Benefits:
The recipe is quick and simple, and making your own fresh cheese guarantees you know what's in it. No starches or added sugars.

## Cream Cheese

Ingredients:
- 250 ml (1 cup) heavy cream
- 50 g (2 oz) goat cheese
- 2.5 ml (½ tsp) vanilla
- 15 ml (1 Tbsp) maple syrup (optional)

Directions:
Whip cream into stiff peaks. Fold in goat cheese, vanilla and maple butter and continue to whip until fully blended.

Benefits:
You have to enjoy a treat once in a while, so if you can make it yourself then you can carefully control what you're putting in your body. Heavy cream is filling and low in sugar. Goat cheese is higher in minerals and lower in lactose than regular soft cheese. Plus, no processed ingredients.

## Cheesecake

Ingredients:
- 12 eggs, separated
- 250 g ghee or butter
- Buttermilk Ricotta Cheese (see recipe outlined before) or approximately 400 ml of ricotta cheese
- 15 ml (1 Tbsp) vanilla extract
- 70 g stevia

Directions:
Mix egg yolks, butter, cheese, vanilla and stevia. Separately whip 12 egg whites. Fold in egg whites, and ladle into a pie crust (see Flaxcracker Crust, above) and bake 30 minutes at 350°F, 20 minutes at 300°F, 30 minutes at 250°F.

Cautions:
This is a rich and filling cheesecake, so be sure to share.

## Mascarpone Cheese Substitute

Ingredients:
- 500 ml (2 cups) cream
- 125 ml (½ cup) powdered milk
- Juice from 1 lemon

Directions:
Whisk cream then slowly add powdered milk and continue to whisk in. Heat to 180°F very slowly in a pot. Add lemon, mix with spoon, and cool 8 hrs. Strain through cheesecloth and squeeze dry.

## Chocolate Bean Pudding

Ingredients:
- 2 cans (400 ml) black beans, drained and rinsed very well
- 45 ml (3 Tbsp) coconut oil
- 2.5 ml (½ tsp) salt
- 2.5 ml (½ tsp) vanilla
- 1 packet gelatin (optional. If you use gelatin, add up to 500 ml of water to make this a lower calorie option. The texture will become more jelly like.)
- 6–8 dates, pitted (note: substituting with stevia will completely change the flavour)
- 3 heaping Tbsp of cocoa powder

Directions:
Add the pitted dates (add first, if they are at the bottom they will help blend), rinsed black beans, coconut oil, salt, and vanilla and blend on highest setting until very smooth. If using gelatin, add in the gelatin powder and add an additional 2 cups of water. Once blended, add in the cocoa powder afterwards, as this will make it very thick and difficult to blend. Blend until smooth.

There are a lot of variations and substitutions you can make for this recipe. Coconut oil can be substituted with cream (½ cup) or even try one whole avocado. I've added a pinch of mint, and dates can be reduced to lower sugar content or substituted with 30 ml maple syrup or honey. I've even made a version without any black beans, substituting with avocado instead.

Benefits:
This is a dessert, but you can make it healthy as well. Keep the sugar content low, and if you like it with avocado, you will be getting the benefit of the healthy oils. Coconut oil has significant amounts of saturated fat but it's also generally a healthy oil.

## Chocolate Avocado Pudding

Ingredients:
- 125 ml (¼ cup) coconut milk
- 2 avocados
- 60 ml (¼ cup) cocoa powder
- 10 ml (2 tsp) vanilla
- 60 ml (¼ cup) maple syrup
- 2 dates, pitted

Directions:
Blend all ingredients on high speed. This is a variation on the Chocolate Bean Pudding listed before.

Benefits:
Flavanols from cocoa powder. Experiment with substitutes and gradually reduce sugar from this recipe and other recipes in general. Your joints will thank you.

## Condiments

### Pizza Sauce

Serves 4 (enough for 1 large pizza)

Ingredients:
- 156 ml can tomato paste
- Oregano/pizza seasoning, to taste
- 15 ml (1 Tbsp) olive oil
- 80 ml water, as required to thin

Directions:
Mix tomato paste, seasoning and olive oil in bowl. Add water slowly and mix until desired consistency is reached.

Benefits:
I've added such a simple recipe in this book to emphasize the importance and benefit of having condiments, sauces and recipes in general that are simple and made with natural ingredients. While many premixed products will contain cheaper ingredients to reduce the cost, like processed vegetable oils and starches, you can still have the convenience of premade foods, like canned tomato paste, which will usually be a simple and clean one or two ingredient mix, and the control over the oils used, by adding in your own extra virgin olive oil. It's a big step up from some of the cheap, processed, inflammatory oils in many prepared and packaged foods.

## *Pesto*

Ingredients:
- 500 ml (2 cups) *fresh* basil
- 125 ml (½ cup) parmesan cheese, grated
- 125 ml (½ cup) extra virgin olive oil
- 3 garlic cloves
- 1 whole avocado, pitted
- 45 ml (3 Tbsp) hemp hearts (optional)

Directions:
Blend basil, oil, avocado and garlic on high until smooth. Add parmesan and hemp and blend on low speed to retain texture. You can also substitute 1 cup of fresh basil with 1 cup of fresh spinach to add thickness.

Benefits:
The avocado gives those healthy, anti-inflammatory oils. Parmesan is zero lactose and probiotic, and olive oil is anti-inflammatory. Hemp hearts also provide anti-inflammatory oils.

## *Olive Tapenade*

Ingredients:
- 375 ml (1.5 cups) black, pitted olives
- 60ml (¼ cup) extra virgin olive oil
- 5ml (1 tsp) anchovy paste
- 45ml (3 Tbsp) capers
- 30ml (2 Tbsp) fresh parsley
- 3 cloves garlic
- 45ml (3 Tbsp) lemon
- salt/pepper

Directions:
Blend all ingredients on slow speed to maintain the texture of the olives (otherwise, if you blend this too fast or too much it will lose all the pleasant texture and feel like baby food). Excellent both with and without the anchovy.

Benefits:
Oleocanthal from the olives and oil, omega-3 oils from the fish, allicin from the garlic—this is an arthritis super food, and tastes great as a spread too.

## Creamy Crab Dip

Ingredients:
- 125 ml (½ cup) sour cream
- 125 g (½ cup) cream cheese
- 1.2 ml (¼ tsp) seasoning of your choice
- 1 clove garlic
- 15 ml (1 Tbsp) lemon
- 15 ml (1 Tbsp) salt
- dash of pepper
- 250 g crab meat
- 30 ml (2 Tbsp) parsley

Directions:
Blend smooth all ingredients except crab or parsley, then add and blend slowly to maintain texture.

Benefits:
Crab is a lean protein, and garlic provides allicin which could help suppress HLA-B27 in AS.

## Spinach and Artichoke Dip

Ingredients:
- 15 ml (1 Tbsp) extra virgin olive oil
- 80 ml (⅓ cup) shallots
- 250 g (8 cups) fresh spinach
- 250 ml (1 cup) artichoke, marinated
- 125 ml (½ cup) mayonnaise
- 125 ml (½ cup) sour cream (make sure you are using one without cornstarch added!)
- 60 ml (¼ cup) parmesan cheese, grated
- salt and pepper to taste

Directions:
Gently sauté shallots, spinach and artichoke in a healthy, high-heat oil like avocado oil. Blend other ingredients on high first, then add sautéed ingredients on slow speed to maintain texture.

Benefits:
Healthy, anti-inflammatory fats from extra virgin olive oil, probiotics from parmesan, and iron from spinach. Mayonnaise can be healthy too if you make your own and use avocado or olive oil.

## Mustard - Raw With Turmeric

No recipe for this one, but I will recommend this as an anti-inflammatory, low-calorie condiment that is very easy to find off the shelf.

## Ranch Dressing

Ingredients:
- 3 cloves fresh garlic, diced finely
- 1.25 ml (¼ tsp) salt
- 250 ml (1 cup) mayonnaise
- 125 ml (½ cup) sour cream
- 70 ml (¼ cup) fresh chopped parsley
- 30 ml (2 Tbsp) fresh chopped dill
- pinch of thyme
- 5 ml (1 tsp) malt vinegar
- 2.5 ml (½ tsp) pepper
- 125 ml (½ cup) buttermilk, thin if required

Directions:
Blend all ingredients on slow speed to maintain texture.

Benefits:
Allicin from garlic and healthy oils from mayonnaise, if you're using a good quality one.

Cautions:
Always check your sour cream for added starch.

## Sour Cream

Ingredients:
- 125 ml (½ cup) kefir
- 250 ml (1 cup) heavy cream
- 10 ml (2 tsp) lemon juice

Directions:
Partially whip ingredients just enough to thicken. Cover loosely and allow to rest at room temperature overnight.

Benefits:
If you can't find a sour cream that doesn't have cornstarch added, you can always make your own. By using a good quality kefir, with bacteria strains like *Lactobacillus rhamnosus* GG, *Lactobacillus casei* and *Lactobacillus acidophilus*, you can ensure your gut receives healthy bacteria that have been shown to lower inflammation and help heal your gut.

## Macadamia "Ricotta" Cheese

Ingredients:
- 250 ml (1 cup) raw macadamia nuts
- 30 ml (2 Tbsp) freshly squeezed lemon juice
- 70 ml (¼ cup) water
- dash of salt

Directions:
Blend all ingredients on medium speed to maintain some texture.

Benefits:
Macadamias are the ideal nut for arthritis sufferers and specifically for AS; they are high in monounsaturated fat, very low in inflammatory omega-6 oils and very low in starch.

## Olive Spread

Ingredients:
- 250 ml (1 cup) black canned olives, pitted
- 3 cloves fresh garlic
- 15 ml (1 Tbsp) freshly squeezed lemon juice
- 30 ml (2 Tbsp) extra virgin olive oil
- 30 ml (2 Tbsp) parmesan cheese, grated
- 30 ml (2 Tbsp) fresh, chopped parsley

Directions:
Blend all ingredients on low to medium speed for a nicely textured, simple spread.

Benefits:
Try this one for its anti-inflammatory oils.

## Kale Guacomole

Ingredients:
- 2 whole pitted avocado
- 60 ml (¼ cup) diced onion
- 1 clove fresh garlic
- 90 ml (⅓ cup) fresh chopped parsley
- 5 ml (1 tsp) salt
- 10 ml (2 tsp) freshly squeezed lemon juice
- dash of pepper
- 125 ml (½ cup) fresh kale
- 45 ml (3 Tbsp) sour cream

Directions:
Chop and steam kale gently to remove bitterness and oxalic acid content. Blend all ingredients on slow to medium speed.

Benefits:
Healthy oils from avocado, allicin from fresh garlic and nutritious kale make this a healthy, anti-inflammatory option. Consider pairing this with fish to get a synergistic effect with onion and help your body produce some glutathione.

## Garlic Mayonnaise

Ingredients:
- 10 ml (2 tsp) freshly squeezed lemon juice
- 1 egg
- 4 cloves fresh garlic
- 250 ml (1 cup) extra virgin olive oil
- 1.25 ml (¼ tsp) salt, dash of pepper

Directions:
In a blender, mix lemon, egg and garlic. While mixing, very slowly trickle in oil at medium-low speed, then add salt and pepper. You can also substitute half of the olive oil with two tablespoons of ghee for a thicker, richer result. Another variation is to whip 125 ml of heavy cream and fold in with the rest of the ingredients for creamier result and lighter flavour. Even try adding horseradish for a kick. Great on cod or on egg as a hollandaise sauce.

Cautions:

A note on raw eggs in recipes. All eggs are required by the USDA to be pasteurized. I have personally never had issues with raw egg, but food contamination, especially from raw meat, can include *Salmonella*, *Yersinia*, *E. Coli* and *Campylobacter*, the very bacteria that are a concern for reactive arthritis and AS. Use caution.

## Avocado Yogurt Dip

Ingredients:
- 1 whole avocado, pitted
- 250 ml (1 cup) low-sugar yogurt or kefir
- 1 clove fresh garlic
- 30 ml (2 Tbsp) freshly squeezed lemon juice
- 2.5 ml (½ tsp) salt, dash of pepper

Directions:
Blend all ingredients on high speed.

Benefits:
Raw, fresh garlic can have a very sharp taste, but this is the best way to obtain the allicin inside. Blending it in a dip this way can help the medicine go down.

## Salmon Mousse

Ingredients:
- 45 ml (3 Tbsp) cold water
- 5 ml (1 tsp) gelatin
- 250 ml (1 cup) sour cream, starch free
- 125 g (4 oz) smoked salmon
- 15 ml (1 Tbsp) freshly squeezed lemon juice
- 1.25 ml (¼ tsp) salt

Directions:
Stir gelatin into water over medium heat. Separately blend sour cream, salmon and lemon. Add gelatin to blender running on slow speed. Chill before serving.

Benefits:
Omega-3 oils from salmon, and gelatin for glycine, help make this a good arthritis-fighting food.

# ACKNOWLEDGEMENTS

Thank you to my wife Izabela, through her words, and my mom Teresa, through her example, in providing me with the support and encouragement to stubbornly try 100 methods and foods to find the 10 that helped.

Thank you to all those that read my rough and sloppy manuscript and provided me great feedback, especially my brother Andrew, and those with medical knowledge, especially Dr. James Hung, Dr. Kiran Manhas, Jon Collins and Graham MacDonald. Thank you to my publishers and editors in putting it all together.

# GLOSSARY OF ABBREVIATIONS

AS – ankylosing spondylitis

COX-1/COX-2 – cyclooxygenase 1 and 2 enzymes

DMARD – disease-modifying anti-rheumatic drug

IgM – immunoglobulin M antibodies

EOs – essential oils

ESR – erythrocyte sedimentation rate

EBV – Epstein-Barr virus

GI – gastrointestinal

NF-kB – a transcription factor that is involved in signalling inflammation in the body

NSAID – non-steroidal anti-inflammatory drug

PA – physical activity

PsA – psoriatic arthritis

RA – rheumatoid arthritis

RS – resistant starch

ROS – reactive oxygen species, an unstable molecule that contains oxygen and react with and damage cells in the body

SAD – standard American diet

SigA – secretory immunoglobulin A antibodies

SI Joint – sacroiliac joint

SpA – spondylarthritis, group including AS, PsA and RA

TEE – total energy expenditure, the total calories used by the body in a day

TNFα – tumor necrosis factor, alpha

# REFERENCES

A. Ebringer, C. W. (1996). The Use of a Low Starch Diet in the Treatment of Patients Suffering from Ankylosing Spondylitis. *Clinical Rheumatology, 15. Suppl. 1*, pp. 62-66.

A. Pallag, G. F. (2018). Equisetum arvense L. Extract Induces Antibacterial Activity and Modulates Oxidative Stress, Inflammation, and Apoptosis in Endothelial Vascular Cells Exposed to Hyperosmotic Stress. *US National Library of Medicine, National Institutes of Health*, PMID 29636839.

A1., E. (1992, Feb). *Ankylosing spondylitis is caused by Klebsiella. Evidence from immunogenetic, microbiologic, and serologic studies.* Retrieved from KickAS.org - The largest Ankylosing Spondylitis support site on the Web!: https://www.ncbi.nlm.nih.gov/pubmed/1561397

al., M. F. (2015, April 15). *Antimicrobial activity of essential oils of cultivated oregano (Origanum vulgare), sage (Salvia officinalis), and thyme (Thymus vulgaris) against clinical isolates of Escherichia coli, Klebsiella oxytoca, and Klebsiella pneumoniae.* Retrieved from US National Library of Medicine, National Institutes of Health: https://www.ncbi.nlm.nih.gov/pmc/articles/PMC4400296/

al., M.-l. e. (2020). Fasting inhibits aerobic glycolysis and proliferation. *Nature Communications*, 1-17.

Alan Goldhamer, D. (1997, Nov 1). *Arthritis and Joint Pain*. Retrieved from CNS: http://nutritionstudies.org/arthritis-joint-pain/

Alqareer A1, A. A. (2006, Nov). *The effect of clove and benzocaine versus placebo as topical anesthetics*. Retrieved from US National Library of Medicine: https://www.ncbi.nlm.nih.gov/pubmed/16530911

AM1., F. (2009, Nov 10). *Modulation of inflammatory disease by inhibitors of leukotriene A4 hydrolase*. Retrieved from US National Library of Medicine: https://www.ncbi.nlm.nih.gov/pubmed/19876785

AP1., S. (2002, Oct). *The importance of the ratio of omega-6/omega-3 essential fatty acids*. Retrieved from US National Library of Medicine: https://www.ncbi.nlm.nih.gov/pubmed/12442909

B Combe 1, P. G. (1996, Jul). *Sulphasalazine in psoriatic arthritis: a randomized, multicentre, placebo-controlled study*. Retrieved from National Library of Medicine, National Center for Biotechnology Information: https://pubmed.ncbi.nlm.nih.gov/8670601/

B Li, C. B. (1994, Oct 3). *Antithetic relationship of dietary arachidonic acid and eicosapentaenoic acid on eicosanoid production in vivo*. Retrieved from National Library of Medicine, National Center for Biotechnology Information: https://pubmed.ncbi.nlm.nih.gov/7852864/

Bioconcepts. (2018, Sep 1). *Ankylosing Spondylitis*. Retrieved from Conditions / Musculoskeletal System: https://www.bioconcepts.com.au/conditions/18/36)

Blancas-Flores G1, A.-A. F.-M.-P.-S.-R.-G.-D. (2012, Aug 15). *Glycine suppresses TNF-α-induced activation of NF-κB in differentiated 3T3-L1 adipocytes.* Retrieved from US National LIbrary of Medicine: https://www.ncbi.nlm.nih.gov/pubmed/22732655

Brianna Elliot, R. (2017, Oct 28). *Does Too Much Vitamin C Cause Side Effects?* Retrieved from Healthline: https://www.medscape.com/viewarticle/825349

C Lawrence Kien, c. a. (2005, Aug 8). *Increasing dietary palmitic acid decreases fat oxidation and daily energy expenditure.* Retrieved from US National Library of Medicine, National Institutes of Health: https://www.ncbi.nlm.nih.gov/pmc/articles/PMC1314972/

Carrillo-Vico A1, R. R.-M. (2006, May). *The modulatory role of melatonin on immune responsiveness.* Retrieved from US National Library of Medicine: https://www.ncbi.nlm.nih.gov/pubmed/16729718

Catherine R. Marinac, 1.,. (2015, Aug 25). *Frequency and Circadian Timing of Eating May Influence Biomarkers of Inflammation and Insulin Resistance Associated with Breast Cancer Risk.* Retrieved from US National LIbrary of Medicine: https://www.ncbi.nlm.nih.gov/pmc/articles/PMC4549297/

Cavallini, J. (2018, April 16). *How-virus-behind-kissing-disease-may-increase-your-risk-autoimmune-diseases-lupus.*

Retrieved from ScienceMag, Science: http://www.sciencemag.org/news/2018/04/how-virus-behind-kissing-disease-may-increase-your-risk-autoimmune-diseases-lupus?utm_campaign=news_daily_2018-04-16&et_rid=383054598&et_cid=1976256

Cerner Multum, Inc. (2018, Aug 29). *What Is Lactobacillus Rhamnosus GG?* Retrieved from Everyday Health: https://www.everydayhealth.com/drugs/lactobacillus-rhamnosus-gg

Charles Piller, J. Y. (2018, Jul 5). *Hidden conflicts? Pharma payments to FDA advisers after drug approvals spark ethical concerns.* Retrieved from American Association for the Advancement of Science: http://www.sciencemag.org/news/2018/07/hidden-conflicts-pharma-payments-fda-advisers-after-drug-approvals-spark-ethical

Charles, E. O. (2003). *Virtual Chembook.* Retrieved from Starch - Iodine: http://chemistry.elmhurst.edu/vchembook/548starchiodine.html

Chris Kresser, M. (2019, May 28). *HLA-B27 and Autoimmune Disease: Is a Low-Starch Diet the Solution?* Retrieved from Chris Kresser: https://chriskresser.com/hla-b27-and-autoimmune-disease-is-a-low-starch-diet-the-solution/

Clarke, C. (2020, July 21). *The Ketogenic Diet and Insulin Resistance.* Retrieved from ruled.me: https://www.ruled.me/the-ketogenic-diet-and-insulin-resistance/

Collado A1, G. J.-G. (1994, Mar 23). *Serum IgA anti-Klebsiella antibodies in ankylosing spondylitis patients from Catalonia.* Retrieved from US National Library of Medicine: https://www.ncbi.nlm.nih.gov/pubmed/8016581

*C-Reactive Protein Test.* (2018). Retrieved from Mayo Foundation for Medical Education and Research (MFMER): http://www.mayoclinic.org/tests-procedures/c-reactive-protein/basics/definition/prc-20014480

Cyrus Khambatta, T. K. (2018). *High-Protein Diets Impair Insulin Sensitivity Despite Weight Loss.* Retrieved from Mastering Diabetes LLC: https://www.masteringdiabetes.org/high-protein-diets-impair-insulin-sensitivity/

Dawn, L. (2012, Sep 26). *The Health Consequences of Too Much Protein.* Retrieved from Happy & Raw: https://www.happyandraw.com//the-health-consequences-of-too-much-protein/

Dona L. Wong, a. T.-F. (2009, Aug 6). *ADRENERGIC RESPONSES TO STRESS: TRANSCRIPTIONAL AND POST-TRANSCRIPTIONAL CHANGES.* Retrieved from US National Library of Medicine: https://www.ncbi.nlm.nih.gov/pmc/articles/PMC2722431/

Ebringer, A. (1989, Aug). *The relationship between Klebsiella infection and ankylosing spondylitis.* Retrieved from US National Library of Medicine: https://www.ncbi.nlm.nih.gov/pubmed/2670258

Ebringer, A. (1992, Feb). *Ankylosing spondylitis is caused by Klebsiella. Evidence from immunogenetic, microbiologic, and serologic studies.* Retrieved from US National Library of Medicine: https://www.ncbi.nlm.nih.gov/pubmed/1561397

Ebringer, A. (2012). *Ankylosing Spondylitis and Klebsiella.* New York: Springer.

F HALTER, A. T. (2001, Sep). *Cyclooxygenase 2—implications on maintenance of gastric mucosal integrity and ulcer healing: controversial issues and perspectives.* Retrieved from US National Library of Medicine, National Institutes of Health: https://www.ncbi.nlm.nih.gov/pmc/articles/PMC1728453/

Fabrizio Cantini, 1.,. (2017, Jun 1). *Risk of Tuberculosis Reactivation in Patients with Rheumatoid Arthritis, Ankylosing Spondylitis, and Psoriatic Arthritis Receiving Non-Anti-TNF-Targeted Biologics.* Retrieved from NCBI US National Library of Medicine, National Institutes of Health: https://www.ncbi.nlm.nih.gov/pmc/articles/PMC5474286/

Fritsche, K. L. (2015, May 6). *The Science of Fatty Acids and Inflammation.* Retrieved from US National LIbrary of Medicine, National Institutes of Health: https://www.ncbi.nlm.nih.gov/pmc/articles/PMC4424767/

Fritsche, K. L. (2015, May). *The Science of Fatty Acids and Inflammation.* Retrieved from US National Library of Medicine, National Institutes of Health: https://www.ncbi.nlm.nih.gov/pmc/articles/PMC4424767/

Gallagher, J. (2018, Sep 6). *Probiotics labelled 'quite useless'.* Retrieved from BBC News: https://www.bbc.com/news/health-45434753

Gallagher, S. (2016, July 14). *Moderately reducing calories in non-obese people reduces inflammation.* Retrieved from TuftsNow: https://now.tufts.edu/news-releases/moderately-reducing-calories-non-obese-people-reduces-inflammation

Garner, R. (2006). *Conscious Health.* Namaste Publishing.

Gianfranca Carta, E. M. (2017, Nov 8). *Palmitic Acid: Physiological Role, Metabolism and Nutritional Implications*. Retrieved from US National Library of Medicine, National Institutes of Health: https://www.ncbi.nlm.nih.gov/pmc/articles/PMC5682332/

H Ahsan, A. A. (2003, Mar). *Oxygen free radicals and systemic autoimmunity*. Retrieved from US National Library of Medicine: https://www.ncbi.nlm.nih.gov/pmc/articles/PMC1808645

Hardman, W. E. (2014, Jun). *Diet components can suppress inflammation and reduce cancer risk*. Retrieved from US National Library of Medicine: https://www.ncbi.nlm.nih.gov/pmc/articles/PMC4058555/

Hardman, W. E. (2014, Jun). *Diet components can suppress inflammation and reduce cancer risk*. Retrieved from US National Library of Medicine: https://www.ncbi.nlm.nih.gov/pmc/articles/PMC4058555/

Hardman, W. E. (2014, Jun). *Diet components can suppress inflammation and reduce cancer risk*. Retrieved from US National Library of Medicine: https://www.ncbi.nlm.nih.gov/pmc/articles/PMC4058555/

HealthDay. (2017, June 24). *Review links conjugated linoleic acid supplementation to CRP*. Retrieved from Medicalxpress: https://medicalxpress.com/news/2017-06-links-conjugated-linoleic-acid-supplementation.html#jCphttps://medicalxpress.com/news/2017-06-links-conjugated-linoleic-acid-supplementation.html

Herron, J. G. (2015, May 9). *Glycine, One Of The Most Important Inflammation Regulators*. Retrieved from The Gut Health Protocol: http://www.theguthealthprotocol.com/wp/glycine-the-most-important-inflammation-regulator/

Hisham M Mehanna, c. a. (2008, Jun 28). *Refeeding syndrome: what it is, and how to prevent and treat it*. Retrieved from US National Library of Medicine: https://www.ncbi.nlm.nih.gov/pmc/articles/PMC2440847/

Hoffman-La Roche, Enbrel Canada Inc, AbbVie Corporation, Bristol-Myers Squibb Canada, Janssen Inc, Pfizer Canada Inc,. (2015, 2016, July 12, Jun 2, Oct 19, April 7, Aug 8, Sept 15, Dec 10). *Actermra, Product Monograph, CIMZIA Product Monograph, Humira Product Monograph, Orencia, Product Monograph, Simponi Product Monograph, Xeljanz Product Monograph, Stelara Product Monograph*. West Sussex, UK: Hoffman-La Roche, Enbrel Canada Inc, AbbVie Corporation, Bristol-Myers Squibb Canada, Janssen Inc, Pfizer Canada Inc,.

Hui-Chun Yu, M.-C. L.-Y.-l.-Q.-B.-S. (2016, Jan). *Sulfasalazine Treatment Suppresses the Formation of HLA-B27 Heavy Chain Homodimer in Patients with Ankylosing Spondylitis*. Retrieved from US National Library of Medicine: https://www.ncbi.nlm.nih.gov/pmc/articles/PMC4730291/

Ippokratis Pountos, T. G. (2012, Jan 4). *Do Nonsteroidal Anti-Inflammatory Drugs Affect Bone healing? A critical analysis*. Retrieved from US National Library of Medicine National Institutes of Health: https://www.ncbi.nlm.nih.gov/pmc/articles/PMC3259713/

J Braun, J. Z.-P. (2006, Apr 10). *Efficacy of sulfasalazine in patients with inflammatory back pain due to undifferentiated* spondyloarthritis and early ankylosing spondylitis: a multicentre randomised controlled trial. Retrieved from US National Library of Medicine: https://www.ncbi.nlm.nih.gov/pmc/articles/PMC1798286/

J H Vaughan, M. D. (1995, Mar 1). *Epstein-Barr virus-induced autoimmune responses. II. Immunoglobulin G autoantibodies to mimicking and nonmimicking epitopes. Presence in autoimmune disease.* Retrieved from US National Library of Medicine National Institutes of Health: https://www.ncbi.nlm.nih.gov/pmc/articles/PMC441471/

J Zochling, D. v. (2005, Aug 26). *Current evidence for the management of ankylosing spondylitis: a systematic literature review for the ASAS/EULAR management recommendations in ankylosing spondylitis.* Retrieved from US National Library of Medicine: https://www.ncbi.nlm.nih.gov/pmc/articles/PMC1798100/

J. Thompson, R. M. (1996). Arthritis: Everything You Need to Know (Your Personal Health). Key Porter Books; 1 Edition.

J.V. Martino, J. L. (2017, May). *The Role of Carrageenan and Carboxymethylcellulose in the Development of Intestinal Inflammation.* Retrieved from US National Library of Medicine, National Institutes of Health: https://www.ncbi.nlm.nih.gov/pmc/articles/PMC5410598/

James T. Rosenbaum, M. a. (2011, Nov 1). *Hypothesis: Time for a gut check: HLA B27 predisposes to ankylosing spondylitis by altering the microbiome.* Retrieved from US National Library of Medicine: https://www.ncbi.nlm.nih.gov/pmc/articles/PMC3204318/

Javier A. Bravo, P. F. (2011, September 20). *Ingestion of Lactobacillus strain regulates emotional behavior and central GABA receptor expression in a mouse via the vagus nerve*. Retrieved from Proceedings of the National Academy of Sciences of the United States of America: https://www.pnas.org/content/108/38/16050

Jean-Michel Gaullier, J. H. (2004, Jun). *Conjugated linoleic acid supplementation for 1 y reduces body fat mass in healthy overweight humans*. Retrieved from National Library of Medicine, National Center for Biotechnology Information: https://pubmed.ncbi.nlm.nih.gov/15159244/

José Francisco Zambrano-Zaragoza, *. J.-C.-R.-A.-P. (2013, Jul 21). *Ankylosing Spondylitis: From Cells to Genes*. Retrieved from US National Library of Medicine: https://www.ncbi.nlm.nih.gov/pmc/articles/PMC3736459/

José Francisco Zambrano-Zaragoza, *. J.-C.-R.-A.-P. (2013, July 21). *US National Library of Medicine National Institutes of Health*. Retrieved from Ankylosing Spondylitis: From Cells to Genes: https://www.ncbi.nlm.nih.gov/pmc/articles/PMC3736459/

Kasa, A. G. (2016, Jun 23). *Evaluation of antibacterial activity of honey against multidrug resistant bacteria in Ayder Referral and Teaching Hospital, Northern Ethiopia*. Retrieved from US National Library of Medicine: https://www.ncbi.nlm.nih.gov/pmc/articles/PMC4919268/

Katri Peuhkuri, N. S. (2012, Jul 20). *Dietary factors and fluctuating levels of melatonin*. Retrieved from US National Library of Medicine, National Institutes of Health: https://www.ncbi.nlm.nih.gov/pmc/articles/PMC3402070/

Ki Won Lee, H. J. (2005). *Role of the conjugated linoleic acid in the prevention of cancer.* Retrieved from National Library of Medicine, National Center for Biotechnology Information: https://pubmed.ncbi.nlm.nih.gov/15941017/

Ki-Jo KIM, C.-S. C. (2012). Anemia of Chronic Disease in Ankylosing Spondylitis: Improvement Following Anti-TNF Therapy. *Archives of Rheumatology,* Issue: Volume 27 - Issue 2 - Page 090-097, https://www.archivesofrheumatology.org/full-text/454. Retrieved from https://www.archivesofrheumatology.org/full-text/454

Kurtoglu E1, U. A. (2003, Dec). *Effect of iron supplementation on oxidative stress and antioxidant status in iron-deficiency anemia.* Retrieved from US National Library of Medicine: https://www.ncbi.nlm.nih.gov/pubmed/14716090

Lee YH1, B. S. (2012, Jul). *Omega-3 polyunsaturated fatty acids and the treatment of rheumatoid arthritis: a meta-analysis.* Retrieved from US National Library of Medicine: https://www.ncbi.nlm.nih.gov/pubmed/22835600

Levine ME1, S. J.-A. (2014, Mar). *Low protein intake is associated with a major reduction in IGF-1, cancer, and overall mortality in the 65 and younger but not older population.* Retrieved from US National Library of Medicine: https://www.ncbi.nlm.nih.gov/pubmed/24606898

Li B1, B. C. (1994, Oct). *Antithetic relationship of dietary arachidonic acid and eicosapentaenoic acid on eicosanoid production in vivo.* Retrieved from US National Library of Medicine: https://www.ncbi.nlm.nih.gov/pubmed/7852864

Liu JF1, L. Y. (2013, Apr). *The effect of almonds on inflammation and oxidative stress in Chinese patients with type 2 diabetes mellitus: a randomized crossover controlled feeding trial.* Retrieved from US National Library of Medicine: https://www.ncbi.nlm.nih.gov/pubmed/22722891

M A Zulet, A. M. (2005, Sep 6). *Inflammation and conjugated linoleic acid: mechanisms of action and implications for human health.* Retrieved from National Library of Medicine, National Center for Biotechnology Information: VL: https://pubmed.ncbi.nlm.nih.gov/16440602/

M Hvatum†, L. K. (2006, Sep). *The gut–joint axis: cross reactive food antibodies in rheumatoid arthritis.* Retrieved from US National Library of Medicine: https://www.ncbi.nlm.nih.gov/pmc/articles/PMC1860040/

M Hvatum†, L. K. (2006, Sep). *The gut–joint axis: cross reactive food antibodies in rheumatoid arthritis.* Retrieved from US National Library of Medicine: https://www.ncbi.nlm.nih.gov/pmc/articles/PMC1860040/

Manninen, A. H. (2004, Dec 31). *Metabolic Effects of the Very-Low-Carbohydrate Diets: Misunderstood "Villains" of Human Metabolism.* Retrieved from US National Library of Health: https://www.ncbi.nlm.nih.gov/pmc/articles/PMC2129159/

Maria Fournomiti, 1. A. (2015, Apr 15). *Antimicrobial activity of essential oils of cultivated oregano (Origanum vulgare), sage (Salvia officinalis), and thyme (Thymus vulgaris) against clinical isolates of Escherichia coli, Klebsiella oxytoca, and Klebsiella pneumoniae.* Retrieved from US National Library of Medicine: https://www.ncbi.nlm.nih.gov/pmc/articles/PMC4400296/

Mark P. Mattson, D. B. (2014, Nov 25). *Meal frequency and timing in health and disease*. Retrieved from Proceedings of the National Academy of Sciences of the United States of America: http://www.pnas.org/content/111/47/16647

Merckoll P1, J. T. (2009). *Bacteria, biofilm and honey: a study of the effects of honey on 'planktonic' and biofilm-embedded chronic wound bacteria*. Retrieved from US National Library of Medicine: https://www.ncbi.nlm.nih.gov/pubmed/19308800

MJ1., F. (1997, Nov). *Protein: metabolism and effect on blood glucose levels*. Retrieved from US National Library of Medicine: https://www.ncbi.nlm.nih.gov/pubmed/9416027

Nicholas J Sheehan, M. F. (2004, Jan). *The ramifications of HLA-B27*. Retrieved from US National Library of Medicine: https://www.ncbi.nlm.nih.gov/pmc/articles/PMC1079257/

Nicholas J Sheehan, M. F. (2004, Jan). *The ramifications of HLA-B27*. Retrieved from US National Library of Medicine: https://www.ncbi.nlm.nih.gov/pmc/articles/PMC1079257/

O'Connor, B. S. (2013, Jul 18). *NSAID therapy effects on healing of bone, tendon, and the enthesis*. Retrieved from US National Library of Medicine National Institutes of Health: https://www.ncbi.nlm.nih.gov/pmc/articles/PMC3764618/

P L Schwimmbeck 1, M. B. (1988, Dec 23). *Molecular mimicry between human leukocyte antigen B27 and Klebsiella. Consequences for spondyloarthropathies*. Retrieved from

National Library of Medicine: https://pubmed.ncbi.nlm.nih.gov/2462350/

P W Wiesenfeld, U. S. (2003, Jun 4). *Flaxseed increased alpha-linolenic and eicosapentaenoic acid and decreased arachidonic acid in serum and tissues of rat dams and offspring.* Retrieved from National Library of Medicine, National Center for Biotechnology Information: https://pubmed.ncbi.nlm.nih.gov/12738189/

Patty W Siri-Tarino, Q. S. (2010, Mar). *Saturated fat, carbohydrate, and cardiovascular disease.* Retrieved from US National Library of Medicine: https://www.ncbi.nlm.nih.gov/pmc/articles/PMC2824150/

Peart, K. N. (2015, February 16). *Anti-inflammatory mechanism of dieting and fasting revealed.* Retrieved from Yale News: https://news.yale.edu/2015/02/16/anti-inflammatory-mechanism-dieting-and-fasting-revealed

Pergolizzi JV Jr1, T. R., & Group., N. R. (2018, Jun). *The role and mechanism of action of menthol in topical analgesic products.* Retrieved from US National Library of Medicine: https://www.ncbi.nlm.nih.gov/pubmed/29524352

Pietro Manuel Ferraro, M. C. (2015, Oct 14). *Total, Dietary, and Supplemental Vitamin C Intake and Risk of Incident Kidney Stones.* Retrieved from US National Library of Medicine, National Institutes of Health: https://www.ncbi.nlm.nih.gov/pmc/articles/PMC4769668/#:~:text=Ingested%20vitamin%20C%20is%20partly,of%20calcium%20oxalate%20stone%20formation.&text=In%20a%20metabolic%20study%20in,oxalate%20excretion%20by%20about%2022%25.

Pontzer, H. (2015). Constrained Total Energy Expenditure and the Evolutionary Biology of Energy Balance. *American College of Sports Medicine*, pp. Vol. 43, No. 3, pp. 110-116.

Qinghui Mu, 1. J. (2017, May 23). *Leaky Gut As a Danger Signal for Autoimmune Diseases*. Retrieved from US National Library of Medicine National Institutes of Health: https://www.ncbi.nlm.nih.gov/pmc/articles/PMC5440529/

R I Sperling, A. I. (1993, Feb). *Dietary omega-3 polyunsaturated fatty acids inhibit phosphoinositide formation and chemotaxis in neutrophils*. Retrieved from US National Library of Medicin: https://www.ncbi.nlm.nih.gov/pmc/articles/PMC288002/

R I Sperling, A. I. (1993, Feb). *Dietary omega-3 polyunsaturated fatty acids inhibit phosphoinositide formation and chemotaxis in neutrophils*. Retrieved from US National Library of Medicine: https://www.ncbi.nlm.nih.gov/pmc/articles/PMC288002/

R. Horwitz, D. M. (2010). Integrative Rheumatology. In D. M. R. Horwitz, *Integrative Rheumatology*.

Rankin, L. (2013, May 15). *Can You Think Yourself Well?* Retrieved from Health: http://www.health.com/health/article/0,,20698923,00.html

Reiko Nagasaka 1, C. C. (2007, May 7). *Anti-inflammatory effects of hydroxycinnamic acid derivatives*. Retrieved from National Library of Medicine: https://pubmed.ncbi.nlm.nih.gov/17499610/

Reilly T. Enos, J. M. (2013, Jan 5). *Influence of dietary saturated fat content on adiposity, macrophage behavior, inflammation, and metabolism: composition matters.* Retrieved from US National Library of Medicine, National Institutes of Health: https://www.ncbi.nlm.nih.gov/pmc/articles/PMC3520521/

Rhodes, K. K.-D. (2015, December 21). *Grapiprant: an EP4 prostaglandin receptor antagonist and novel therapy for inflammation.* Retrieved from Wiley Online Library: https://onlinelibrary.wiley.com/doi/full/10.1002/vms3.13

Rhodes, K. K.-D. (2015, Dec 21). *Grapiprant: an EP4 prostaglandin receptor antagonist and novel therapy for pain and inflammation.* Retrieved from Wiley Online Library, Veterinary Medicine and Science: https://onlinelibrary.wiley.com/doi/full/10.1002/vms3.13

Ridker PM, E. G. (1990, Aug). *False positive mononucleosis screening test results associated with Klebsiella hepatic abscess.* Retrieved from US National Library of Medicine, National Institutes of Health: https://www.ncbi.nlm.nih.gov/pubmed/2371976

RL1., V. (2004, Mar). *The therapeutic implications of ketone bodies: the effects of ketone bodies in pathological conditions: ketosis, ketogenic diet, redox states, insulin resistance, and mitochondrial metabolism.* Retrieved from US National Library of Medicine: https://www.ncbi.nlm.nih.gov/pubmed/14769489/

Robinson, C. (1957, Aug 15). *Emotional Factors and Rheurmatoid Arthritis.* Retrieved from US National Library of Medicine: https://www.ncbi.nlm.nih.gov/pmc/articles/PMC1823975/

S. Hizmetli1, R. A. (2015). *AB0786 Circadian Rhythm of Melatonin in Ankylosing Spondylitis: Correlation with Disease Activity, Quality of Life and Enthesitis Score.* Retrieved from Annals of the Rheumatic Diseases: https://ard.bmj.com/content/74/Suppl_2/1161.3

Sarah L. Gaffen, 1. R. (2015, Sept). *IL-23-IL-17 immune axis: Discovery, Mechanistic Understanding, and Clinical Testing.* Retrieved from US National Library of Medicine: https://www.ncbi.nlm.nih.gov/pmc/articles/PMC4281037/

Senna MK1, O. S.-A. (2012, Nov). *Serum melatonin level in ankylosing spondylitis: is it increased in active disease?* Retrieved from US National Library of Medicine: https://www.ncbi.nlm.nih.gov/pubmed/22057142

Shane M Huebner, J. P.-F. (2010, Aug). *Individual isomers of conjugated linoleic acid reduce inflammation associated with established collagen-induced arthritis in DBA/1 mice.* Retrieved from National Library of Medicine, National Center for Biotechnology Information: https://pubmed.ncbi.nlm.nih.gov/20573944/

Silva J1, A. W. (2003, Dec.). *Analgesic and anti-inflammatory effects of essential oils of Eucalyptus.* Retrieved from US National Library of Medicine: https://www.ncbi.nlm.nih.gov/pubmed/14611892

Solutions, A. (2018). *C-Reactive Protein.* Retrieved from MedlinePlus Trusted Health Information for You: https://www.nlm.nih.gov/medlineplus/ency/article/003356.htm

Steven A. L. W. Vanhoutvin, F. J. (2009, Aug 25). *Butyrate-Induced Transcriptional Changes in Human Colonic*

*Mucosa*. Retrieved from PLOS One: https://journals.plos.org/plosone/article?id=10.1371/journal.pone.0006759

Steven DiLauro, M. a.-C. (2011, August 1). *Ileitis: When It Is Not Crohn's Disease*. Retrieved from US National Library of Medicine, National Institutes of Health: https://www.ncbi.nlm.nih.gov/pmc/articles/PMC2914216/

Taha Rashid, 1. C. (2013, May 27). *The Link between Ankylosing Spondylitis, Crohn's Disease, Klebsiella, and Starch Consumption*. Retrieved from US National Library of Medicine: https://www.ncbi.nlm.nih.gov/pmc/articles/PMC3678459/

Tathagat. E. Waghmare*, H. B. (2014, Jun). *Antimicrobial Properties of the Methanolic Extracts of Zingiber officinale (Ginger) in Escherichia coli and Klebsiella pneumoniae*. Retrieved from www.academia.edu, IOSR Journal of Pharmacy and Bilogical Sciences: http://www.academia.edu/7050392/Antimicrobial_Properties_of_the_Methanolic_Extracts_of_Zingiber_officinale_Ginger_on_Escherichia_coli_and_Klebsiella_pneumoniae

Thomas A Perry, X. W. (2021, Jan 27). *Association between current medication use and progression of radiographic knee osteoarthritis: data from the Osteoarthritis Initiative*. Retrieved from National Library of Medicine, National Center for Biotechnology Information: https://pubmed.ncbi.nlm.nih.gov/33502488/

U.S. Department of Health & Human Services. (2009). *The Energy Metabolism Project*. Retrieved from National Institute on Aging: https://www.nia.nih.gov/research/labs/lns/energy-metabolism-project

UC Davis Health. (2000, Dec 1). *UC DAVIS STUDY SHOWS SPIRULINA BOOSTS IMMUNE SYSTEM*. Retrieved from UCDavis Health: https://www.ucdmc.ucdavis.edu/publish/news/newsroom/2658

V Srinivasan, 1. G. (2005, Nov 29). *Melatonin, immune function and aging*. Retrieved from US National Library of Medicine: https://www.ncbi.nlm.nih.gov/pmc/articles/PMC1325257/

V.R. Windor, J. (1987, June). *Hyper-responsiveness to EBV in ankylosing spondylitis*. Retrieved from US National Library of Medicine, National INstitutes of Health: https://www.ncbi.nlm.nih.gov/pmc/articles/PMC1002175/?page=1

*WebMD*. (2018). Retrieved from What is a C-Reactive Protein Test?: http://www.webmd.com/a-to-z-guides/c-reactive-protein-crp

Weil, D. A. (2018). *Elevated C-Reactive Protein (CRP)*. Retrieved from Drweil.com: htts://www.drweil.com/health-wellness/body-mind-spirit/heart/elevated-c-reactive-protein-crp/

Wikipedia. (2018, Nov 9). *Gram-Negative Bacteria*. Retrieved from Wikipedia - The Free Encyclopedia: https://en.wikipedia.org/wiki/Gram-negative_bacteria

Wikipedia. (2018, Nov 9). *Klebsiella pneumoniae*. Retrieved from Wikipedia - The Free Encyclopedia: https://en.wikipedia.org/wiki/Klebsiella_pneumoniae#frb-inlinc

Yeager, A. (2020, September 14). *Immune Cell and Its Cytokine Control Exploratory Behavior in Mice*. Retrieved from The Scientist: https://www.the-scientist.com/news-opinion/immune-cell-and-its-cytokine-control-exploratory-behav ior-in-mice-67930?utm_campaign=TS_DAILY%20 NEWSLETTER_2020&utm_medium=email&_hsmi =95275118&_hsenc=p2ANqtz-_wjR7rELDrL8vr9b6 BbiueYrkhKF8XSPZp0ywghwm0bW2RVfRXmPz

Yun-Hee Youm, 1. K. (2015, Mar 21). *Ketone body β-hydroxybutyrate blocks the NLRP3 inflammasome-mediated inflammatory disease.* Retrieved from US National Library of Medicine: https://www.ncbi.nlm.nih.gov/pmc/articles/ PMC4352123/

Zhao S1, C. H. (2017, Nov 31). *The association of NLRP3 and TNFRSF1A polymorphisms with risk of ankylosing spondylitis and treatment efficacy of etanercept.* Retrieved from US National Library of Medicine: https://www.ncbi. nlm.nih.gov/pubmed/28116820

Zhong Z1, W. M. (2003, Mar). *L-Glycine: a novel antiinflammatory, immunomodulatory, and cytoprotective agent.* Retrieved from US National Library of Medicine: https://www.ncbi. nlm.nih.gov/pubmed/12589194

Printed in Great Britain
by Amazon